MIRACLES

OR

"I HAVE NO MORE BOILS"

Patrick Massey MD PhD MhD

Contact information:
Patrick Massey MD PhD MhD
1544 Nerge Rd.
Elk Grove Village IL 60007
www.alt-med.org

Library of Congress Control Number
ISBN 978-0-9981986-0-6

Illustrations by Christine Benhart

DEDICATION

Nothing in this world happens without the help and inspiration of others. It is one of the wonderful ways in which we are all connected. I give thanks to my wife Daryl and to my children (by age) Ryan, Katelyn, Jasen, and Nathan for putting up with my many peculiarities, sharing fantastic journeys and discoveries, and keeping me grounded enough that I have stayed on this plane lo these many years. I give many thanks to their profound and innate wisdom and creativity that has been a driving force in this book's evolution.

I give thanks to my parents Onie and Joyce whose lives they shared with me have shaped mine in more ways than I could have possibly imagined.

Many thanks to those who when I asked (often) for inspiration and direction, they answered in great measure.

I am constantly amazed at how the universe brings people into our lives when we need them. The wonderful illustrations are the brainchildren of the talented graphic artist Christine Benhart. She is the daughter of my longest friend John (I met when we were five years old) and his wonderful wife Diane.

I thank my "brother from another mother" Brad Mehr whose encouragement for over a two year span during our regular coffee at Starbucks helped bring this book to fruition I am also indebted to my physician friend and another "brother from an another mother," Kevin Matthews MD, for his guidance, time, and effort in critically reviewing this book.

Contact Information

Patrick Massey MD PhD MhD

c/o ALT-MED Medical and Physical Therapy

1544 Nerge Rd

Elk Grove Village IL 60007

Office: (847) 923-0046

Office web site: alt-med@msn.com

Book web site: patrickmasseymiracles.com

Table of Contents

"Every affliction has a remedy.

Those who persistently seek

answers will ultimately find

them and be transformed by this

alchemic process."

Patrick B. Massey MD PhD MhD

INTRODUCTION

Welcome, my brothers and sisters, to the 21st century. According to the science fiction stories there should be flying cars, regular vacation tours surfing the rings of Saturn, we should be living hundreds of years, and all illnesses and diseases long eliminated. Well, this certainly is an exciting new age but there are no flying cars or surfing vacations to Saturn, and I doubt my IRA would last me hundreds of years. Regrettably, illness and disease are more prevalent now than ever before. However, this is the 21st century and there are answers waiting to be discovered.

> *"At the center of our being you have the answer; you know who you are and you know what you want."*
>
> **Lao Tzu**

Illness and disease are not unknown to us. Every new age of man has its biblical-level pestilences that challenge that age. In Europe during the Middle Ages it was the black plague. Most of the evidence points to the bacteria *Yersinia pestis* as being the causative agent and transmitted to humans by fleas. Although the people of that time discovered that concoctions such as "thieves oil" and "four thieves vinegar" offered some protection against the plague (they may have been effective flea repellants) they eventually discovered that improvements in sanitation and personal hygiene as well as the establishment of quarantine zones for those infected were the determining factors in limiting further spread of the disease. Three hundred and fifty years later societal changes ushered in by the industrial age created the perfect conditions for the epidemic spread of tuberculosis. One of the societal changes was the rapid population shift from farms and small towns to the cities. As a result, people were nutritionally challenged and lived in squalid, overcrowded conditions. They were at the greatest risk of not only contracting the disease but of rapidly dying from it. During the industrial age, tuberculosis (*Mycobacterium tuberculosis)* spread rapidly and just as quickly killed over one third of those infected. By the end of the 19th century it was estimated that 80 percent of the population of the United States had been exposed to and possibly infected with tuberculosis before their twentieth birthday. As in the case of the plague, people rose to the occasion and discovered that improvement in sanitation and nutrition, and isolation of those infected (tuberculosis sanitaria), were the most effective remedies. It would be a long time before the discovery of an effective antibiotic.

In this new age I feel that chronic illness is our biblical-level pestilence. There might be some disagreement since cancer or heart disease by themselves could be considered a plague of modern times. Alzheimer's disease, diabetes and many other illnesses could justifiably also be considered as contenders for this dubious title. As serious as these individual illnesses are they all share one common trait. They are all defined as chronic illnesses. Just as our ancestors found solutions for their biblical level plagues now is the time to unearth the answers to the chronic illnesses of our age. As someone who has suffered for a decade from the affliction of chronic pain (but no longer), I know the frustration and anger, indeed even to the point of despair, of not finding solutions within the traditional and nontraditional medical systems. Imagine the level of my exasperation considering I am a physician with one foot in traditional medicine and the other in nontraditional medicine. The overwhelming fatigue that comes from persistent failure, fear, and disappointment were at one time my most unwelcome and unrelenting companions. From my studies and experiences I have concluded that the solution to chronic illness cannot be found exclusively in medications, machines, supplements, or therapies. The answer lies within each of us.

When I found no substantive answers for my own chronic pain by looking outside of myself, the only place left to go was inside. It was there I began to identify for myself, and ultimately for my patients, those secrets of healing practiced by the ancient miracle healers and known to the spectacular healers of today. I realized that, for the most part, we are perfect and that within our very being is everything we need to heal. Also within us are the causes for most of our chronic illnesses. In order to heal we must become be cognizant of the fact that we are both the creator of our chronic illnesses as well as the architect of our health. Through awareness, acceptance of personal responsibility, and force of will, cures can be attained. The road may be long and it is not always easy. There are many stumbling blocks with no guarantee of complete success. In spite of all that, answers await those who are ready. What will be gained are profound transformations, personal growth, and a greater freedom from chronic illness. From my perspective, it is a trip well worth the effort.

Health could be defined as freedom and independence from a state of illness. The historical progress of humankind has always been toward greater degrees of freedom and has consisted of many steps, more forward and some backward, toward self-determination. This can be seen as humankind has progressed from a state of near slavery, with no independence and very little personal responsibility, led by benevolent or often not so benevolent rulers to increasing degrees of emancipation and expansion of personal responsibility. The same is true in health. We are evolving from reliance on the absolute authority of physicians and the medical system to one of questioning and independent thought and action. We are becoming bold enough to really rock the boat, and indeed this boat needs some serious rocking. Just as the squalid environment of the Middle Ages enabled the flea-borne plague and the crowded living conditions of the industrial revolution created the perfect storm for tuberculosis, we have designed the ideal environment for chronic illness to flourish. We, like our ancestors, have the ability to modify that design to one that encourages health.

I have always had an affinity for the healing arts. Studying and understanding the healing process seems to be deeply embedded in my DNA. Although my father was a career soldier and I spent my early years on military bases, at the ripe old age of four, dressed in a child-sized military uniform, my father's commanding officer asked me if I was going to enlist in the Air Force like my father. To his and my father's amazement I clearly replied that I was going to be a doctor. I simply knew. When I was accepted into medical school I envisioned myself as the heroic surgeon saving lives in the nick of time by the sharp edge of a scalpel. This was not to be my path. As I progressed through my medical career I saw and physically felt the suffering of those with chronic illnesses especially those who had been marginalized by the medical system because of the "incurability" of their illnesses. I felt great frustration that more could not be done for these unfortunate people. Rather than go into the lucrative, procedure-based medical specialties I searched for a medical career in which I could help (teach) patients to find their way through chronic illness. I found integrative medicine. For the past thirty years most of my medical practice has consisted of treating patients with chronic illnesses from Alzheimer's disease to acne and everything in between including pain, depression, anxiety, and "just feeling lost." In the thirty years I have been practicing medicine, I realize that chronic illness is the consequence of afflictions not just the body but also of the mind and spirit. Even though medications, supplements, herbs, etc, may improve many of the symptoms of a chronic illness a cure only happens when there is healing also at the level of the mind and spirit. The path to healing is unique. The usual "one-size-fits-all" approach will almost always fail. Each person must discover the specific combination of body, mind, and spirit healing that defines their own path. Even though we are all moving in the same general direction, we are traveling our own individual paths and must listen to our own unique rhythms. I offer this book not as the standard "self-help" program but as a compass to begin to map your individual path toward self-healing and, ultimately, your own miracles.

I would like to be able to say that the first part of the title of this book, *Miracles*, is a reflection of my amazement at the individual transformation possible in the treatment of chronic disease at this time. In part it is but, truth be told, once the book was written I could not think of a good title. Knowing this book was going to be written and published at some time in the future I took a short-cut on uncovering the title. During a meditation I went forward in time and envisioned a copy of the completed book lying on my desk. I simply looked at the front cover of the book and there appeared the word "Miracles". There were other words I could barely make out and did not make sense. Those words became clear because of a statement made by one of my patients. She had traveled to a Central American country and had developed boils over most of her body. Many dermatologists, internists, and infectious disease physicians were unable to help her. Knowing that all the bad and ugly diagnoses had been ruled out by her physicians, I suspected some alteration in her bowel bacteria from her travels and suggested a change in diet. After a month, I saw her again and the first sentence that passed from her lips was "I have no more boils." I thought those are the words of the rest of the title to my book.

Miracles

Chapter 1

These are Changing Times

M ay you live in interesting times is a timeworn Chinese saying. This aphorism, however, is not considered a positive catchphrase. It is meant as a curse for one's enemies hoping that the world around them would be disordered and turbulent. It seems that this misfortune has been bestowed on all of us. We are indeed living in "interesting times." Our world is changing faster now than any time in

> *"Chronic illness, like health, is a personal choice. Both require a conscious effort."*
>
> **Patrick Massey MD, PhD**

history. In the past societal changes were measured in decades or even centuries. Today our sense of society is upended about every three to five years. It seems that if you simply oversleep on the weekend, civilization will have passed you by. For many it may feel like we are powerless in the face of such rapid change, that we are like the leaves subjugated to the more powerful forces of a tornado. This is especially evident in American health care. *"May you live in interesting times,"* and indeed we do.

Over the past fifty years advances in modern medicine have been fast and furious. Robotic and laser surgery, artificial limbs, genetic manipulation, nanotechnology and more are no longer the dreams of science fiction. Indeed these technologies used in medicine today did not even exist when I started medical school in 1982. As in many science fiction novels, one would also assume that, with such an advanced medical system, chronic illness would be uncommon. In sharp contrast, people in the United States have never been sicker, requiring an ever increasing number of medications, medical tests, therapies, surgery, money, and other resources. In 2015, it was estimated that the direct and indirect medical costs of the seven most common chronic diseases exceeded 1.3 trillion dollars (1, 2). By 2050, this cost is estimated to surpass six trillion dollars per year (3). With the Star Trek-like advances in medicine we should be healthier but we are not. It seems illogical that as medical science has advanced, chronic illness has become more common. We are living longer and there is a valid argument that a longer life increases the risk of chronic illnesses. However, these chronic illnesses are now being manifested in childhood rather than just at an older age.

Most Common Chronic Diseases
- Cancer
- Stroke
- Diabetes
- Lung disease
- Hypertension
- Heart disease
- Mental illness

We were all encouraged by the spectacular successes in medicine like the development of the polio vaccine and medical research in the 1940s-1970s held onto the notion that chronic illnesses would eventually be cured by a pill. I remember being told by my 6th grade science teacher that the cure for the common cold was just around the corner. We must be on the longest street in the history of man because that corner is still a long time coming. Becoming aware of the futility of unearthing miracle "cures," by the 1980s medicine's vision changed from curing chronic illness to simply controlling the symptoms of an illness so that a patient would not die prematurely. Just reducing the symptoms of a chronic illness is not an irrational approach in the short term but it does not correct the underlying reason for the chronic illness. It is like a boat with an open hole in the bottom and the only thing that is done is to continuously pump out the water. The underlying problem is not corrected. The rapidly growing prevalence of chronic illness is forcing to us to realize that the futility of the ever increasingly expensive "disease maintenance" paradigm that pervades modern medicine. We are being ushered (forced?) into a new perception that curing chronic illness is simply beyond the skill of modern medicine. Ultimately we must become the captain of our own ship and accept responsibility for our health. If we are willing to do this, then we can change our destiny.

One thought-provoking development in modern medicine has been the evaporation of the patient's responsibility for their health. Less than one hundred years ago it was expected that a person took care of them-selves and when that failed then it was the physician and medical system to the rescue. Today, however, it is believed by many that the current healthcare system is supposed to take care of you cradle to grave. Like "helicopter parents," physicians, nurses, therapists, and other health care providers are supposed to be available 24/7 and constantly monitoring for the slightest changes. If you are not compliant with your medications, it is a failure of the physician and nurse. If you are not doing prescribed physical therapy exercises, it is the therapists who are not doing their jobs. Billions of dollars have been spent on medical monitors and computer applications all designed to minimize any personal responsibility. This is especially evident with the explosion of electronic devices and applications designed to remind us to exercise, take medications, and even sleep. Even with these advances, the clinical result of a poor lifestyle is not really your fault because living a healthy lifestyle is too "hard" in the modern world. Everyone is too busy to get enough sleep, exercise, follow a reasonable diet, and reduce their stress. Besides, many symptoms of chronic illnesses can be easily suppressed by a plethora of powerful and expensive medications. If the symptoms of a chronic illness are minimized then everything is fine and no changes are needed. I remember a specific patient who was taking seven different medications tell me in absolute honesty that he felt he was in good health because he had no symptoms of his chronic illnesses. Further eroding the importance of personal responsibility and good lifestyle choices, modern medicine would have you believe that chronic illness is the result of "bad" genes or some set of undefined and unfortunate circumstances. Once a chronic illness has been diagnosed, it falls into the classification of a perpetual condition over which you have little or no control. Blaming the genes is simply a "get out of jail free" card for the medical system, and the treatment of the chronic illness fibromyalgia is a perfect example. In modern medicine we have no idea what it is or what causes it, and medications are not particularly effective, so we look for a genetic excuse to explain our impotence. Fate rolled the dice and you came up "snake eyes." No one is to blame. Just accept your circumstances, take you medications and move on. However, this is a time of great change.

Lifestyle decisions are indispensable in order to reverse course in chronic illness. These decisions require a desire to change and the effort to bring this change to fruition. Desire, effort, and consistency over time are the components of personal responsibility. Lifestyle changes require ongoing education and support of the patient. Education takes time, effort, money, and a one hundred percent commitment by the patient. Alcoholics Anonymous is a well-known example of a successful program that supports its members, while emphasizing personal responsibility and commitment (4, 5). In stark contrast, the modern medical system, both traditional and nontraditional medicine, does not require significant participation by the patient. The medical system believes that it is more efficient and cost effective to prescribe a drug, supplement, herb, therapy, or surgery rather than do the hard work involved with consistently encouraging exercise, sleep, stress reduction, and dietary changes. Indeed there are powerful forces trying to maintain the status quo. As I was once told by a top hospital executive, money is made by treating illness, not creating health. For example, insurance companies, with a high turnover of customers, do not want to invest any money promoting healthy lifestyle changes in their customers in case another insurance company will benefit from their efforts. The government and medical societies give lip service to lifestyle changes but do little to stress the importance of prevention so there is little progress in this area and people suffer. Yet there is robust medical research spanning centuries that strongly correlates the origins of many chronic illnesses with lifestyle choices. One could surmise that our choices about our lifestyle not only predispose us to chronic illness but that we and our lifestyle choices have the potential for a greater impact on our health than any aspect the current medical system. Only we have the capacity to effect the substantial change needed to change our destiny. If we choose a life of stress, sleep deprivation, a lack of exercise, poor food choices, tobacco, alcohol, and legal and illegal drugs, there is an increased risk of high blood pressure, heart disease, cancer, diabetes, Alzheimer's disease, etc. If chronic illness is a roll of the dice then the dice are loaded by personal choice. To a considerable extent nature, our own evolution, and the ever-increasing cost of medical care are forcing us to realize that we are the exclusive architects of our health, good or bad. We need to embrace a new understanding of why chronic illness occurs and how to reverse it—not simply manage it but actually reverse it. This new understanding must take into account the reality that for most chronic illness everything you need to be healthy is already inside of you. That begins by your realization that YOU are both the primary cause and solution to most of your health issues. Truly this is a time of great change.

The new path to health begins by delving into the wisdom of the past. For thousands of years and in many cultures it has been a common realization that we are composed of a combination of a body, a mind, and a spirit. Without these three fundamental elements we cannot exist as we do in the physical world. We have known for centuries that thoughts and feelings such as fear, happiness, contentment, and turmoil have a significant impact on the development of chronic illness. Feelings and sometimes thoughts are how the spirit communicates with the mind and these communications can then be born into the physical world through the body. Our experiences and the results of our decisions manifested through the body, in this case health vs. illness, serve as an educational tool for the mind and spirit prompting better lifestyle choices. The interactions between the body, mind, and spirit are reflected in our lifestyle choices and ultimately our health. Understanding how the body, mind, and spirit interact is crucial to making good lifestyle choices and ensuring long-term health. With a greater knowledge of how the body, mind, and spirit collaborate, long-term health is not only possible but readily achievable by everyone. This discovery refuses to wait for modern medicine to catch up. It is happening now in over a thousand different ways and the results are miraculous.

Chapter 2

Why Does Chronic Illness Still Exist?

In order to understand why chronic illness still exists we first need to define illness. There are two expressions of all illnesses, acute and chronic. "Acute" refers to an illness that happens suddenly, without the necessity of a specific underlying disease. "Chronic" identifies a disease process that develops over time. The common causes of acute illness are infections, toxins, and trauma. Some may argue that a first heart attack or asthmatic attack is acute but, in truth, they are the result of a series of long-standing, non-fatal physiologic changes culminating in the presentation of chest pain and shortness of breath respectively. The reason that a chronic illness is not immediately evident is that the body is able to compensate to some degree for the changes in the state of health. When the body can no longer compensate, the symptoms of the chronic illness are manifest.

> "*Miraculously recover or die. That's the extent of our cultural bandwidth for chronic illness.*"
>
> **S. Kelley Harrell**

Chronic illness is the enduring traveling companion of humanity and today it is riding "shotgun", head out the window, hair flowing the wind, and loudly singing "Smoke on the Water." It is large and in charge. Eighty percent of all medical care is consumed in the treatment of chronic illness. Like a giant swarm of indestructible cockroaches, no matter the effort, we just cannot get rid of this pestilence. Medicine has been fighting chronic illness for a long time but we keep forgetting what we have learned. The historical record dating back millions of years to our earliest known ancestors are replete with examples of the physical result of chronic illness. Human remains from ancient cultures often show the wear and tear of life—arthritis, diabetes, parasite infestations, heart disease and even cancer—but not to the extent of chronic illness today. Interestingly the cultures of the ancient world in Europe, Asia, Australia, Africa, and the Americas all developed and used effective medical therapies for relief of the physical symptoms of chronic illnesses. Many of the ancient therapies for chronic illnesses such as diabetes, asthma, and various bowel conditions were reasonably effective. Some may have been as effective in suppressing the symptoms of an illness as prescription medications today. Therapies developed healing, and the use of various minerals and herbs were so effective that they are still in use today! There is an increasing amount of published research in the medical literature demonstrating their benefits. Although healers in the ancient world prescribed herbs and therapies to limit the symptoms of chronic illness, there is ample evidence that they understood the importance of lifestyle choices and recommended specific changes in diet, exercise, and even stress reduction. Almost 2,500 years ago the Greek physician Hippocrates (460-370 BCE) taught that illness was not the result of whimsical decisions of the gods or bad luck (no dice throwing here) but the result of lifestyle choices and environment. Interestingly Hippocrates, one of the most important influences of Western medicine, would be considered quite the alternative practitioner by today's medical standards. One of the reasons why chronic illnesses are so prevalent today is, in part, that humanity often forgets what it has learned. As a result, the medical community is deluded into believing that the medical therapies and lifestyles of antiquity are primitive, based on superstition, and generally ineffective even in the face of overwhelming evidence to the contrary. As everything moves full circle old medical knowledge and health concepts are being re-discovered. If these re-discoveries were left to the laborious pace of medical research it would take centuries. People do not want to wait that long and are increasingly taking an active role in the treatment of their chronic illnesses.

Another case in point about lifestyle choices and health can be found in comparing our modern diet to those dietary practices of the ancient world. Our modern diet is the brainchild of the United States Department of Agriculture (USDA). The first USDA nutrition guidelines were published in 1894 by Dr. Wilbur Olin Atwater strongly advocating for more variety, proportionality, moderation, and concentration on nutrient-rich foods and less starch and sugar (6). These dietary recommendations seem like sound advice and are consistent with many time-tested culturally-based diets.

In 1992 the guidelines changed reflecting the ever-increasing influence of special interest groups of the grain, meat, and dairy industries. As with many governmental agencies tasked with protecting the health of the citizens, special interests triumphed over science and became the new standard. As the government-approved standard found its way into medical schools, nursing schools, and dietary education programs, it polluted entire generations of front-line health care providers. With such an extreme emphasis on grains and starch, Louise Light (designer of the first food

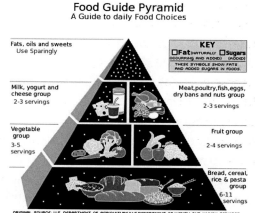

pyramid) warned that such a diet could lead to an epidemic of obesity and diabetes (7), and she was right. For over twenty years national nutritional recommendations followed the starch heavy food pyramid, and now it is not surprising that obesity and diabetes are epidemic across all ages and ethnic groups in the U.S. Unfortunately, obesity and diabetes seems to be the United States number-one export to the rest of the world. In stark contrast culturally-based diets are healthier and, in the case of the

Mediterranean diet, have been demonstrated to prevent and even improve the symptoms of several chronic illnesses like high blood pressure and type II diabetes (8, 9). The realization of the direct relationship between diet and chronic illness is not new. The link between a poor diet and chronic illness has been recognized for thousands of years but has been ignored, dismissed, or forgotten by modern medicine. What really drives this point home is the overall quality of most hospital food. A selection of food that is strongly associated with contributing to chronic illness is the very same food offered to people who are critically ill and desperately trying to recover. In stark contrast, many of the dietary rules found in Judaism and Islam may have originated with health benefits in mind. In Islam, a halal diet forbids the consumption of certain foods including meats and animal products containing or exposed to blood. Using a strict, standardized butchering process, halal meats probably would have fewer parasites and bacteria when compared to other butchering methods in use before modern technology. In Judaism, food preparation is also very important. The preparation of meats, dairy products, and eggs is exacting and reduces the risk of parasitic and bacterial infestation of food. In antiquity, non-kosher foods probably would have been high in parasites, viruses, and bacteria. Making diet and the preparation of food a matter of religious edict would have ensured the improved health and survival of a large population. Many religions also impose fasting during certain times of the year and accumulating medical research is confirming that there are substantial health benefits to intermittent fasting for obesity, diabetes, heart disease, and perhaps cancer. Through the centuries we discovered the benefits of herbs, diet, exercise, meditation, stress reduction, and even sleep. With all that we have learned over the ages one should ask, "Why does chronic illness even exist?" The answer is mind-numbingly simple. We choose it.

The expression of chronic illness requires three specific conditions: a lifestyle detrimental to good health, an illness that is at least non-fatal in the early stages, and enough time for the illness to overwhelm the body's ability to compensate for the imbalance(s) caused by of the illness. However there is no guarantee that a chronic illness will germinate from the seed of a physically unhealthy lifestyle. Other powerful influences are needed and these influences come from the mind and spirit. No one is perfectly healthy for their entire life. Through the continuous interactions of the body, mind, and spirit, everyone will, eventually, develop some medical condition. It might be mild and not require medical intervention but it could also result in life-threatening symptoms compelling heroic measures to secure life. Unfortunately the incidence of serious, life-threatening chronic illness is on the rise. To put the impact of chronic disease in perspective, it affects over 50 percent of the U.S. population with an alarming increase in frequency in childhood and accounts for more than 80 percent of all medical costs (10). Even though chronic illness seems to be inevitable, much of it is preventable and in many cases curable.

One could postulate that chronic illness exists because of the consequences of "cause and effect." After all, it is commonly believed that "cause and effect" is the nature of all things and it is. "Cause and effect" implies that chronic illness is the direct result of a series of poor lifestyle choices (cause) and the resultant physical and mental deterioration (effect). If a person eats poorly, never exercises, and has unrelenting stress, then heart disease, cancer, high blood pressure, obesity, diabetes, and strokes are sure to follow. It is simple "cause and effect." When studying the incidence of chronic illness in a large population, the principle of cause and effect seems to be an indisputable fact. When Americans follow the traditional 1992 food pyramid, fail to exercise, and fill their days with unrelenting stress then obesity, heart disease, depression, and diabetes are the direct repercussions. However, at the level of the individual, "cause and effect" is less obvious. I have treated many people who have made a lifetime of healthy choices and still develop serious, chronic illness. There are others, who seem to be masters in the art of making poor lifestyle decisions, even living a life of debauchery, and chronic illnesses give them a wide berth and generally they are quite healthy. One patient comes to mind who has a history of smoking a pack of cigarettes per day for fifty years, serious drug and alcohol use, tremendous stress, sleep deprivation, and poor diet. After all this, at the age of seventy, the patient's only medical issue is a "touch" of emphysema. In contrast, I also have patients who have strictly adhered to a healthy lifestyle and still develop heart disease, diabetes, Alzheimer's disease, and even cancer. One patient was a lifelong strict vegan, never smoked or drank alcohol, held a low stress job, did not live in a toxic environment, and had no family history of cancer. Yet she developed an aggressive form of colon cancer. I know that my experiences are not unique; other physicians have experienced the same profound incongruities in their medical practice. Over the past five decades, a mountain of medical research has been collected trying to explain the risk factors for chronic illnesses including the roles of gender, lifestyle, and especially genetics. Although there are tantalizing trends in discovering genetic risk factors for developing a specific chronic illness, except for specific, well-defined genetic diseases, it cannot be said with certainty whether a individual person with an increased genetic risk will or will not develop a specific chronic illness. This suggests that a complex interplay of factors, both known and unknown are necessary for the expression of a serious chronic illness. For this reason, the simple "cause and effect" model described earlier cannot clearly predict whether health or chronic illness will be the final outcome for any individual. Chronic illness to a degree may be determined by a physical "cause and effect" relationship but other influences, specifically those of the mind and spirit, are significantly more impactful. In the development of chronic illnesses the complex interactions between the mind and spirit eclipse the straightforward physical "cause and effect".

What is occurring in the world now is that each person is realizing that they have the potential to become a creator of miracles and this is no more evident than in the health field. We cannot depend on the current medical system to cure chronic disease. It simply is not designed to do that (explained in later chapters). Each patient must become the creator of their own health. Many of my patients have traveled long and far in the traditional and non-traditional medical systems before ending up at my door. It is not uncommon for them to say to me that they are hoping for a miracle. I often tell them that I can help but that they are the creator of their own miracles.

IT'S ALL IN THE GENES

Jointly, in 1962, James Watson, Francis Crick, and Maurice Wilkins received the Nobel Prize for their work in determining the molecular structure of deoxyribonucleic acid (DNA) (11). DNA is found in the nucleus of most of our cells. Mature red blood cells of most animals do not have a nucleus. DNA is made up of many smaller components called genes. Genes carry the information each cell needs for the assembly and functioning of our physical being. Genes are composed of repeating series of four molecules called nucleotides. These nucleotides are composed of a molecule of guanine, adenine, thymine, or cytosine, all with a sugar (monosaccharide) and a phosphate group attached. These repeating sequences of nucleotides act like a biologic Morse code. The dots and dashes in Morse code represent letters of the alphabet and unique sequences of nucleotides act like the dots and dashes coding for specific genes. Genes are the key to our genetic make-up and are the blueprint for our physical form. That discovery opened the door for the hypothesis that genes may be the root cause of all chronic illnesses. In 1990, the Human Genome Project undertook the incredible task of sequencing the entire human DNA (over three billion nucleotide pairs). In 2003, this effort was declared "complete" with the fully realized sequencing of the human genome, and the project discovered that humans have about twenty-one thousand genes which is more than a chicken but less than a grape (11, 12). One of the goals of this effort was to determine if one or more genes would be consistently associated with a specific chronic illness. Even before the sequencing of the human genome, we knew that there were rare chronic illnesses caused by a defect in a single gene. It was postulated that defective genes might be important in the expression of other chronic illnesses. Examples where a physical alteration in a single gene reliably and directly causes a specific illness include sickle cell anemia resulting from a mutation changing hemoglobin structure making the red blood cells very stiff (12). Stiff red blood cells get stuck in small blood vessels causing oxygen deprivation and severe pain. This illness increases the risk of death from infections and stroke. Another chronic illness, cystic fibrosis, occurs through a mutation in the enzymes that regulate how water and salt move out of cells. These defective genes have a great impact on how the cells of the lungs, intestine, and pancreas function (13). Those with cystic fibrosis are at a substantial increased risk of pneumonia, malabsorption of nutrients, and diabetes. Tay-Sachs disease is caused by a gene mutation on the fifteenth chromosome (14). This mutation causes a build-up of toxic fats in the brain. Children with Tay-Sachs often die within four years even with the best medical care. In sharp contrast to the aforementioned rare chronic illnesses, what the Human Genome Project discovered was that many different genes are only modestly associated with an increased risk of a single chronic illness such as heart disease, diabetes, and dementia. Some researchers hoped that the Human Genome Project would demonstrate that chronic illness is the result of a limited number of "bad" genes. Based on this premise, a chronic illness would be just bad luck and there would be little that you could ever do to prevent or reverse it. Therefore, chronic illness would be predetermined by your genes no matter what your lifestyle, and this simply is not the case. Correlation does not prove causation and, to a large extent, our lifestyle choices determine if "good" or "bad" genes are expressed. For the most part, genes play a secondary role in the development of chronic illness.

IT'S NOT JUST IN THE GENES

The hypothesis that changes in the DNA are the primary reason for the expression of chronic illness is complicated by the reality that just having genes associated with a chronic illness does not mean that the chronic illness will be manifest. Recent and robust medical research has discovered that the expression of genes can be influenced by both lifestyle choices and by even by thought itself.

Epigenomics is the study of how a cell regulates the expression of its genes (15). Specific molecular (epigenetic) modifications of the genes by the cell itself can create a healthy cell or turn a healthy cell into cancer. These molecular modifications in the genes are not inheritable traits. They are the result of the effect of the environment (lifestyle). This means that two identical cells can have completely different destinies depending on their environment. A parent's lifestyle can affect the expression of genes and not just for that person but also for their offspring, even spanning several generations. Even though parental genes are not altered, that tendency of a cell to modify the expression of a gene in either a positive or negative manner seems to pass from parent to offspring. It would thus seem accurate to say "The sins of the father are to be laid upon the children." (16) As an example, if a female mouse is chronically exposed to the chemical bis-phenol A (BPA) it alters how the mouse's cells modify the expression of the genes without changing the genes themselves. The result of these gene modifications is obesity. Imagine an epigenetic modification is the gear shift on a car but the car is the gene. The car can be put in either forward or reverse dramatically changing the direction of the car without affecting the car itself. This change in how the genes are expressed is also seen in the offspring even without BPA exposure. If the parent is stuck in reverse the offspring will also be stuck in reverse. BPA is used as a plastics hardener. It is often contained in the lining of food cans and hard plastics like pipes and some plastic bottles. It would be safe to say that most of us are regularly exposed to BPA, and probably has contributed to obesity reaching epidemic levels in the United States. Interestingly female mice exposed to BPA in conjunction with a specific "detoxification" diet birth normal, non-obese mice. Lifestyle decisions are critical.

Despite what I learned in my numerous biochemistry classes, we are not just a rucksack of chemicals interacting in some random manner. We are much more wondrous and complex. Most people would agree with the idea that we are composed of not just a body in a physical sense but also of a mind that occupies both a physical (brain) and energetic space (thoughts). Many, though not all, would also maintain that we also have an energetic spirit. So we are a three- or at least two-layered being which exists simultaneously in two different worlds, the physical and the energetic. Although chronic illnesses are expressed in the physical body it is commonly realized that they also are also associated with changes in mentation, cognition, and mood, and therefore affect the mind. The effects of chronic illness on the spirit are subtler. They may be expressed as despondence, melancholy, and a profound feeling of loneliness and/or disconnectedness. The interactions between the body, mind, and spirit are integral to both the development and the cure of chronic disease.

Our health is the result of the interplay between our body, mind, and spirit. The interactions between all three facets of our humanity determine whether or not we are healthy. Medical research has revealed that mental/spiritual practices like meditation can have a direct effect on our DNA and the expression of specific genes. In some studies the genes associated with inflammation and chronic pain can be turned off by the practice of mind-spirit therapies such as meditation. These mind-spirit activities do not just reduce the chemicals of inflammation but actually turn off those genes instrumental in creating the inflammation (17 - 19). Other studies show that meditation has the potential to physically alter DNA to the point of increasing lifespan (20, 21). Our DNA and genes are important, but my brothers and sisters, through interactions between the body, mind, and spirit, we are both the primary cause of and miraculous solution to our chronic illnesses. After millions of years of evolution we have finally arrived at a point where we are increasingly responsible for all of our actions and their results, both good and bad. We are capable of transforming chronic illness into health. As Hippocrates said, "*Natural forces within us are the true healers of disease.*" We are all now quite capable of performing all the wonderous miracles we will ever need.

Miracles

Chapter 3

The Roots of Chronic Illness

When looking for the root cause of most chronic illnesses the answer is not too far away. The root cause of most chronic illnesses is us. There often are mitigating and contributing factors that influence the severity of the chronic illness but we are the primary cause. Most of us come into this world with a healthy body very much in balance, a body that according to some estimates should last for almost two hundred years. Yet in the industrialized nations the average lifespan is less than half of

> *"Diseases of the soul are more dangerous and more numerous than those of the body."*
>
> Cicero

that. Moreover, if we calculate how many years we actually are in good health-that is not requiring any medications-that estimate is maybe half of the average lifespan, about forty years. Currently in the United States, the years of good health may be even fewer, as chronic illnesses such as diabetes, high blood pressure, and heart disease are now at epidemic levels in younger adults and, frighteningly, are happening at much earlier ages in children, promoted by a rapid rise in obesity, decrease in physical activity, quality of food, and increased stress. Even the best-built machine will fail unless it is well looked after and regular maintenance is done.

The common denominator in all chronic illnesses is you. If you are in excellent health physically, mentally, and spiritually, it would be unexpected that any illness could establish a lasting foothold. If you are not in good health-physically, mentally, and spiritually-then many illnesses can easily become established, lead to further weakening, and open the door wider for the expression of life-threatening illnesses. Once one illness establishes a foothold, it often lays the ground-work for a cascade of more serious illnesses. For example, chronic stress often precedes high blood pressure. High blood pressure promotes coronary artery disease and coronary artery disease is a primary cause of a heart attack and/or stroke. This process is like a row of dominos. When one starts to fall, the rest effortlessly follow suit. Stress elevates the blood pressure leading to small tears in the walls of the arteries. The body repairs these tears by using cholesterol, much like wall spackle, filling in the torn areas of the artery. This is the beginning of arterial plaque. Over time, if the stress and high blood pressure are not addressed the tears become bigger, needing more cholesterol and leading to a dangerous buildup of often unstable plaque. Ultimately a piece of the plaque may break off (a simplification of an incredibly complex process and I apologize to my cardiology brothers and sisters). This wandering piece of plaque can obstruct a critical artery to the heart or brain causing a myocardial infarction (heart attack) or stroke. Who is at fault for this series of unfortunate events? The body certainly isn't. It is totally blameless in the evolution of this process. The body is doing the best it can and is responding exactly as it should. It is incapable of doing otherwise. The responsible party(s) for unfortunate outcome lies uniquely within the domains of the mind and spirit. Yet the medical standard of care is aimed, almost entirely, at the physical expression of the illness with blood pressure and cholesterol-lowering drugs. There is little comprehension of the root cause-that first falling domino deeply embedded in the mind and spirit. That is the reason why chronic illness rarely heals. The reason for a chronic illness is rarely the fault of the body. Chronic illness's many roots go much deeper. They have their origins in the mind and spirit.

Ever since the discovery of DNA, it was speculated that all chronic illnesses could be the result of bad genes. Identifying the genes responsible for creating a specific chronic illness would usher in a new age of medical therapy and healing. When the entire human genome (DNA) was finally decoded it was hoped that the information that came from this heroic effort would yield great insight into the genetic cause of all illnesses. The result could lead to the development of genetically targeted drugs, therapies, and even genetic manipulation that would finally end our long and tempestuous relationship with chronic illness, ushering in a new age of "super" humans who would be resistant to most illnesses. On the other hand, what followed was quite sobering. It was discovered that many different genes were associated with but not specifically causative for any chronic illness. These genes needed to interact both with other genes as well as the environment in specific and complex ways for the development of a chronic illness. Even more confusing was that those genes and combination of genes associated with a specific chronic illness were not consistent between individuals. Even an illness as common as high blood pressure could involve many different sets of genes in each individual. To date there are at least twenty-nine different genes associated with an increased risk of high blood pressure. However simply possessing the genes for high blood pressure does not guarantee that an elevation in blood pressure will be manifested. Individually each gene minimally increases the risk of high blood pressure but the interactions between the genes can dramatically increase the risk especially in an environment conducive to high blood pressure. That is to say that the pathway to a specific chronic illness may vary widely between individuals, and even with the individual, depending on environment. Those with the genes increasing the risk of high blood pressure may never develop high blood pressure if they regularly reduce their levels of stress perhaps by meditating or exercising on a regular basis. In contrast, the same individuals working at an unrelentingly high stress job, with no exercise or stress-relieving practice such as meditation, probably will develop high blood pressure.

Targeting specific genes with a genetically designed drug is, given today's technology, impossible (and probably futile). Imagine trying to find a medication that could target twenty nine different genes, with these genes varying among individuals. Even if it were possible, the cost would be prohibitive to all but the ultra-wealthy, and maybe prohibitive even to them. To make it even more complex, the proteins encoded by these "bad" genes may be necessary for life. Proteins made by any of our genes have many functions in human physiology, not just promoting a chronic illness like high blood pressure. There is a term for this call "protein moonlighting." This discovery was first published in 1988 by Piatigorsky, O'Brien, Norman, et al. (22). As a result, altering or suppressing these "bad" genes could have significant, unforeseen serious health consequences. What this means is that there are substantial limits to the "linear" cause-and-effect approach to chronic illness held in such high esteem by traditional and much of nontraditional medicine. Modern medicine has made some giant steps in clarifying and classifying chronic illness states and in developing and refining the technology used in treating the symptoms of many chronic illnesses. These technological breakthroughs are rivaling the medical technology of our best science fiction. Modern medicine still falls short of curing chronic illness because of the linear thinking that pervades most medical thought. Although a cause-and-effect approach is extremely effective in the emergency room (My hand is bleeding because I cut it-the cause; it is bleeding-the effect; it needs stitches-the applied medical therapy), it is a woefully inadequate process of thinking in the treatment of chronic illnesses. As an active member of both the traditional and nontraditional the medical communities I can state with confidence that our understanding of the origins of chronic illness is still quite rudimentary. American psychologist Abraham Maslow once said, *"I suppose it is tempting, if the only tool you have is a hammer, to treat everything as if it were a nail."* Maslow's statement indicates that a single mindset cannot correct all problems and the current medical approach to chronic illness is pretty hammer-intensive. I would paraphrase Maslow's words this way; *"If the only tool you ever use is a hammer, everything WILL be treated as a nail."* We need more sophistication in our therapeutic options than just a hammer. Fortunately within each of us are all of the tools and sophistication we need, including the occasional hammer, for most chronic illnesses.

A person is composed of three parts-a physical body, the physical and energetic mind, and an energetic spirit. All contribute, in some fashion, to establishing either a state of health or chronic illness. The physical aspects of a chronic illness are obvious. These symptoms can be easily measured and effectively suppressed with pharmaceuticals, supplements, therapies, and/or surgery. Most of the practice of traditional and nontraditional medicine is laser-focused on eliminating the physical symptoms of an illness because it is easy to measure a result as well as quite effective in preventing premature death. If the physical symptoms of an illness are suppressed, then, in the minds of patients, physicians, health care workers, insurance executives, hospital administrators, government, and many nontraditional practitioners, their work is done. It isn't! Sir William Osler MD (father of American medicine) once said, *"The good physician treats the disease; the great physician treats the patient who has the disease."*

Chronic illnesses related to the mind are more complex to treat than are the physical manifestations of chronic illnesses. They often require a substantial time commitment and personal effort by both the patient and practitioner. Changing the convictions and desires of the mind can be difficult because we all too often become irrationally attached to a specific idea or thought process even if it no longer serves our best interests. The consequences of correcting the faulty thought process can, however, be lasting and life-changing for the patient. A chronic illness whose origins are found in the mind is not synonymous with mental illness, although there can be considerable overlap of symptoms like depression, anxiety, irrational fears, and disturbed sleep. Indeed, these symptoms are so common that they challenge the hypothesis that depression, anxiety, and many other "mental" disorders only arise from some poorly defined physiological imbalance in the brain. Chronic illnesses can be rooted in persistent faulty thoughts or perceptions about oneself or others. Irrational guilt and the inability to forgive oneself are common and persistent faulty thoughts that substantially impede the healing process. The symptoms of these types of chronic illness are not reversed with pharmaceuticals, supplements, or therapies. Although many suffer from these types of chronic illnesses little authentic effort is expended by both traditional and nontraditional medicine in the elucidation of the root cause of the illness and implementation of truly effective treatments.

Spirit-level illness affects both the physical and mental domains; thus, healing at the spirit level can profoundly improve physical and mental health. The root of an illness at this level may stretch back lifetimes, originating in the past, affecting the present, and impacting the direction of the future. This is a territory that almost everyone in traditional and nontraditional medicine avoids at all costs and into which only the exceptional and fearless healer ventures. Yet the physical and mental payoff when healing the spirit can be rapid and complete. Healing at this level can result in what many consider to be true miracles. Without intervention, spiritual-level healing is slow, often taking lifetime, but under the right circumstances (often with guidance) it can seem to be instantaneous. It is possible that cases of spontaneous cures are, in fact, a healing of the spirit. Select bio-energy-based healing techniques can rapidly and profoundly open the door to healing the spirit if the person is open to the process. I personally have experienced the healing of the spirit, and when it finally happened the therapeutic result was so fast as to be practically instantaneous. It was preceded, however, by years of hard work and an abundance of energy-based therapies.

Healing of the spirit is the most impactful level of healing. Life flows from the spirit into the physical realm. Healing the spirit intensely influences the overall health of the mind and body. This level of healing is to a great extent a process of self-forgiveness. Over the millennia the laws of most cultures have been punishment-based. If a person does something outside of the law, punishment is the only road to redemption. Unfortunately even after a debt to society has been paid, the individual continues to be punished by society and/or by self. For many, the "sin" may seem too onerous to ever be forgiven, so the punishment continues and the health of body and mind suffer. It can be almost impossible to convince those punishing themselves to stop, because the punishment is perceived to be payment for an unforgivable sin. There are no medications, supplements, or surgery for this condition. Many are afflicted with this self-destructive process and in my opinion it is a prevailing source of pain and suffering in the world. Only when the person finally opens to the healing of their spirit and experiences the reality of forgiveness of self does integrated healing (body, mind spirit) actually happen. Then miracles are achievable.

HEALING THE BODY

A fifty-year-old, obese male who had rarely done any exercise over his lifetime began to develop knee pain. The pain increased in severity over the years to the point where walking was limited. Neither traditional physical therapy nor a series of steroid injections into the knee space had succeeded in alleviating the pain. One physician even recommended knee replacement. The patient was taking three different pain medications, one stomach medication (to treat the side effects of the pain medications), as well as an antidepressant and sleep aid for his depression over his increasingly poor quality of life. All in all, he was taking nine medications to treat one chronic illness and four medication side effects. I recommended a protocol for modest weight loss and a gradual increase in pain-free physical activity. Once he lost some weight and gradually increased his physical activity through tai chi and swimming, the knee pain improved. He did not need as much of his pain medications and no longer needed the stomach medications. His depression and sleep improved as his quality of life improved. Long-term, the patient continues to do well. He will occasionally take one over-the-counter pain medication for his knees after extended activity. Problem solved and a minor miracle.

HEALING THE MIND

Faulty thoughts are often at the heart of mind-based illnesses. For example, a forty-five-year-old female patient, an overachiever and very successful in business, began to lose interest in most things in life. She had a supportive husband and two fine children. She was financially secure and had no serious illness. The patient, however, grew up in an excessively goal-driven family. For the past five years, the patient had become less satisfied with her life.

Her primary physician diagnosed her with depression and she was started on medications. The initial medication helped her depression a little but she gained fifteen pounds as a side effect. The patient tried a number of other anti-depressants without success. The side effects of other anti-depressants included insomnia, daytime fatigue, decreased libido, and a feeling of being disconnected. In taking the time to talk in depth with the patient, she revealed that she wanted to work less and spend more time with her husband and children—in essence, to stop and smell the roses. Instead, she was dominated by an overwhelming driving need for achievement. She defined her worth by her achievements. Once she realized that this need for achievement was a way of her gaining acceptance and love from her parents, her life changed. Interestingly, it was her mother who instilled in her this fear-driven, unfulfillable need for achievement, with messages such as, "No woman should ever have to depend on a man" and "It is a male-dominated world and a woman needs to fight harder every day." Her fundamental feminine nature had been subjugated by a faulty interpretation of the masculine nature's need for achievement. Once she understood the faulty thoughts that were impacting her life, she realized that she could be a mother and wife as well as successful in business. Her dissatisfaction was that her "feminine" energy was trying to establish a better balance with her "male" energy. Her depression quickly improved and began her own consulting business. She is now her own boss and has more time for family. Currently she is not taking any anti-depressants and is quite happy. This was a moderate miracle.

HEALING THE SPIRIT

A twenty-eight-year-old male presented to my office with a myriad of seemingly unrelated symptoms: nonspecific pain, constipation, insomnia, unsettling dreams, and an inability to have a lasting, monogamous relationship. In his relationships there always was some reason for it to end even if was going well. A common feeling was that the other person was "too good" for him. Medical tests were unremarkable and he was not clinically depressed. In the past, medications, counseling, supplements, and various traditional and nontraditional therapies had proven useless. I was suspicious that the root of his symptoms was not in his body or mind, and suggested that an energy-based therapy termed a past-life regression, looking for the root cause. He was open to the suggestion and the root cause was indeed found. It involved a series of events in several past lives. The decisions he made in those lives resulted in pain and suffering for others. Although he is a very different person in this lifetime, he still could not forgive himself for his past transgressions even though they were quite acceptable during those time periods. Upon realizing and understanding this, he was able to truly forgive himself. Most of his symptoms rapidly melted away over a period of a few weeks. The insomnia and disturbing dreams ended almost immediately. Today he is happily married with a growing family-a major miracle.

Chapter 4

What Happened To The Miracles?

I can say with absolute confidence that by the time we reach adulthood, we have all experienced something extraordinary in our lifetimes. It could be the birth of a child, seeing the Rocky Mountains for the first time or looking up in the night's sky and discovering that luminescent marvel we call the Milky Way. A wondrous event can also be unpretentious like feeling the weight of a snow-flake on your cheek in the crisp early winter morning. All wondrous events expand us. Witnessing or experiencing a miraculous event is one way to connect with a reality beyond our five senses. Although we live in a time of incredible technological

> *"**Miracle**: An effect or extraordinary event in the physical world that surpasses all known human or natural powers and is ascribed to a supernatural cause...or considered as a work of God."*

achievements we have become insensitive to the existence of real miracles. Some are so starved of truly wondrous experiences that they claim it to be a sign of direct divine intervention when the face of some "holy" person is suddenly recognized on a piece of toast or in the shape of a potato chip. What of experiencing healing miracles? Real, "in your face," undeniable miracles of healing by extraordinary healers are vanishingly rare today and when they do happen they are often dismissed. It was not always this way. In the distant past miracles, especially of healing, were so profound that they became the basis of legends.

In ancient times, it seemed that God, or the gods, their messengers, chosen ones, shamans, etc. performed numerous and spectacular wonders or miracles to move the hearts and elevate the minds and aspirations of the masses. Many of these recorded miracles involved healing of chronic illness. These "chosen" healers willingly demonstrated a level of knowledge far beyond what was common in their time. They were seemingly able to bend the very laws of nature and regularly cure the incurable. Legends, and in some cases recorded history, tell us that these "gods," angelic beings, and ancient miracle workers (some say aliens too) walked among men, teaching, educating, and performing these healing miracles. Indeed, they clearly demonstrated extraordinary knowledge and abilities. For example, Hippocrates was well thought of as a great healer in ancient Greece, but another physician, Asclepius, was so good at his craft that the Greeks (and others) considered him a god. We can argue whether these people existed or that miraculous healing actually occurred, but the phenomenon of spectacular healing in the ancient world does not seem to happen today, at least not with the same frequency or of the same magnitude.

According to Homer's *Iliad*, Asclepius was a physician who repeatedly demonstrated his medical prowess while treating the wounded Greek soldiers during the battle of Troy. Greek legends, however, tell us that Asclepius was a demi-god whose father was the Greek god Apollo and mother a mortal Greek woman, Coronis. To make a long story short, Coronis died while pregnant with Asclepius and Apollo delivered his son by performing the first caesarian section. Asclepius was taught the art of healing by a centaur named Chiron. A centaur is a mythological creature 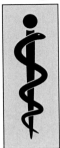 with a human upper body and the lower body of a horse. It is said that Asclepius became a remarkable healer and surgeon and was even able to bring people back from death (which we can do in modern medicine, to a degree). Modern medicine, both traditional and nontraditional, honors the healing ability of Asclepius by using his symbol, a snake wound around a wooden staff, as a symbol of medical knowledge and clinical expertise. Even the symbol for the very conservative *Journal of the American Medical Association* contains the staff of Asclepius. American physicians, upon graduation from medical school, honor Hippocrates by reciting the Hippocratic Oath but acknowledge that Asclepius was a physician of greater significance. The original Hippocratic Oath is thought to begin with, "I swear by Apollo the Physician and by Asclepius the surgeon..." not the Hippocrates or the American Medical Association...Asclepius.

Thousands of years before Asclepius and Hippocrates, there lived an Egyptian healer of note, Imhotep. Most people identify the name Imhotep with movies about ancient Egypt and undead mummies. In the movies he is depicted as a high priest who had a forbidden love with some female member of the royal court. In Hollywood's vivid imagination he was buried alive and condemned to an existence between life and death. The real Imhotep was considerably more interesting. He lived during the Third Dynasty of Egypt (about 2,600 BCE). The name Imhotep means "the one who comes in peace" (people had really cool names in ancient times), and he was considered a physician. He was also a "polymath" or a person who demonstrates a profound proficiency across a wide variety of subjects. Leonardo da Vinci is another example of a polymath. In 2611 BCE, Imhotep was the chief architect of the first step pyramid constructed in Saqqara Egypt for the pharaoh Djoser. He was also a priest, an astronomer, and physician. His full title was Chancellor of the King of Egypt, Doctor, First in Line after the King of Upper Egypt, Administrator of the Great Palace, Hereditary Nobleman, High Priest of Heliopolis, Builder, Chief Carpenter, Chief Sculptor, and Maker of Vases in Chief— quite a resume for one man. As an active physician, Imhotep diagnosed and treated over 200 diseases, including what we believe were tuberculosis, gallstones, and appendicitis. He also was an accomplished surgeon. I am amazed that with all of his responsibilities he actually had time to see patients. Perhaps he had extra time because he was not saddled with all the insurance and governmental paperwork required of modern surgeons. So miraculous were the results of his treatments and therapies that for three thousand years after his death he was worshipped as a god not only in Egypt but in both the Greek and Rome cultures.

According to the Christian bible, over 2,000 years ago Jesus of Nazareth healed the chronically ill and even raised the dead using words as his primary instrument of healing. Many people believe that he was the Son of God and as such felt that he had power over demons, disease, and death. Others regard him as only a prophet of God but still having great powers. Some hold he was only a man. There are others who believe that he did not actually exist but that the story of his life was a compilation of numerous other historical stories. Either way, according to the historical record we have, Jesus of Nazareth was not considered a physician but repeatedly demonstrated a deeper understanding of disease than was commonly known at that time (and even now) and consistently demonstrated miraculous powers of healing. Jesus of Nazarus performed thirty-four recorded miracles. If you assume demonic possession to be a description a chronic illness, twenty-seven miracles (about 80 percent) involved healing chronic illnesses. For most of these miraculous cures the only tool was the vibrational sound of Jesus' voice.

All cultures throughout their history have stories of powerful healers such as the Qigong practitioners of Asia, the Aborigines of Australia, and the Maori of New Zealand. Many stories of uniquely powerful Native American healers (North, Central, and South America) exist today. For Native Americans, without a written language, much of their history has, unfortunately not been recorded, and when written language from Europeans was available, the recording of their history and techniques was actively suppressed by the U.S. government and others. I mention Native

American shamans because their approach to illness is quite complex and, to my understanding is quite complete, involving treating the body, mind, and spirit. It is to be hoped that when they decide to reveal and record their rich medical history this knowledge will be available for the benefit of all mankind.

In modern times there are many famous "miracle" healers. All countries have talented healers but Brazil seems to have the greatest concentration. I cannot vouch for the validity of their healing claims but it seems that many people, world-wide, have benefitted from their expertise. There is some skepticism about

> All cultures have stories of outstanding healers. Not including these stories does not diminish my respect and admiration. It is simply too much for this book.

miracle healers and rightfully so. Not everyone is healed and charlatans abound. I have personally met some very impressive healers whom I can strongly endorse-Rosalyn Bruyere (California), Janice Hayes (Georgia), Wan Su Qian (Beijing, China), Kimberly and Charles Curcio (Georgia). However, as talented as these healers are, their successes do not come close to the successes of the miracle healers of antiquity. Something has changed. Today people with chronic illness cannot depend on the remarkable healers who populated the past to cure their illnesses. These miracle workers of the ancient world either no longer exist or their appetite for publicity has diminished significantly with time. So why don't "big" miracles happen anymore? If someone was regularly curing the incurable and raising the dead I would assume that would be a prime-time news story. I cannot speak for all cultures and peoples, but in general, big healing miracles stopped happening, consistently, about 2,000 years ago.

Although there are many outstanding physicians, researchers, and healers alive today and many life-saving therapies and procedures have been discovered, reliable cures for chronic illnesses are rare. Some might disagree and mention the discovery of the polio vaccine by Jonas Salk MD. His discovery has saved more lives than any of the miracle healers of the past; however, his vaccine prevents polio; it does not treat it once it has become established. I would venture to say that most people alive today do not know who Dr. Salk was and what he did. He also gave his discovery to the world without patent or financial return. In my eyes that action was a moral miracle achieving the level of biblical significance. Even with Salk's great contribution to mankind, I would speculate that, in ancient times, more Egyptians knew of Imhotep and Greeks knew of Asclepius than Americans today know of Dr. Jonas Salk. I personally know many outstanding traditional and non-traditional physicians and healers and yet cannot name one who compares to the miracle healers of the past. Is it possible that the time of "wonder and magic" is over? To some degree I believe that it is, but the greatest of human miracles are happening now.

Over the last half-century or so, almost on a daily basis, we are achieving the miraculous in many aspects of the human condition. Every five years there seems to be an important technological leap redefining our very existence. Even our most mundane experiences today exceed anything of the ancient world. Today, we can travel around the world flying at five hundred miles per hour in a thirty-ton metal tube 30,000 feet above the earth connected to the world via the internet and having a hot meal (in first class). Unfortunately, traveling in coach is significantly less extraordinary. The fact that our airline luggage arrives generally on time, intact and in the right luggage carousel, to me is a miracle in itself. Private companies are working to make space travel as common as flying from Chicago to Los Angeles and NASA safely landed a Volkswagen-sized robot on a planet forty million miles away controlled from a computer on earth. WOW! In the medical field, surgery, aided by robots, can be done on fetuses while still in the womb. Computer chips can be implanted in arteries to monitor the heart's function by cell phone (yes, there is an app for that), and physicians can connect with physicians and patients across the globe as easily as making a phone call. But none of these modern miracles is accomplished by a single person. Rather, it takes many people with incredible training and expertise working together to accomplish the unbelievable. Each person working independently as hard as they could would be inadequate. The miracles of today are not isolated events brought on by single individuals, but are the result of many people sharing a common vision creating many small miracles that coalesce into the fantastic developments we all enjoy. Even though the first moon landing was a momentous event, it could not be claimed by a single person. As Neil Armstrong said, *"That's one small step for man, one giant leap for mankind"* composed of innumerable small miracles.

Some might say that the "Age of Miracles" has ended. I would, however, suggest that the real "Age of Miracles" is just beginning. The miracle is us–all of us. God has never needed to perform individual miracles because He built them into the system, into all of us. We are now at a point in our evolution where we are capable of creating our own health. This means that we all have the ability to self-heal, to transform ourselves physically, mentally, and spiritually. It is absolutely miraculous. Rather than individual, tremendous feats of healing done exclusively by the rare and obviously superior humans of antiquity, what is happening now is that billions of smaller miracles of healing are occurring every day by average persons like you and me. We are discovering and capitalizing on our own inner strength to heal and grow. Similar to advances in technology, the result of many smaller improvements and discoveries, the knowledge from billions of humbler healing miracles are accumulating and causing a profound metamorphosis in our understanding and treatment of chronic illness and, ultimately, our society. That is the true miracle...not to create a world that depends on rare opportunity and the benevolence of the few extraordinary miracle workers but to create a world where everyone actualizes the miracles they want and need. That, my brothers and sisters, is true freedom and has been a discovery over 10,000 years in the making. That is what this book is about. But with freedom comes its close companion, personal responsibility. You are the creator of your miracles and it is you who, on all counts, are responsible for your own health. Albert Einstein was a brilliant man and not just in physics. He was also one bodacious philosopher. He once said, *"There are only two ways to live your life. One is as though nothing is a miracle. The other is as though everything is a miracle."* Not only are we experiencing this new "Age of Miracles", we are actively creating it! Everything IS a miracle.

Chapter 5

The Slow Evolution of Medicine

Sir William Osler MD (1849-1919) was an illustrious Canadian physician and one of the four founders of what is now Johns Hopkins Medical Center. He was recognized by his peers as a phenomenal healer and teacher and so profoundly changed the practice of Western medicine that he is considered to be the father of modern American medicine. He once said, *"The aim of medicine is to prevent disease and prolong life, the ideal of medicine is to eliminate the need of a physician."* He knew that healing does not happen if only the symptoms of an illness are addressed-unfortunately a lesson not well understood by both traditional and nontraditional medicine. Healing happens only when you, the patient, take control and look deeper.

> *"The art of medicine consists in amusing the patient while nature cures the disease."*
>
> Voltaire

The chronic illnesses of today also affected our ancestors, probably just not as often. The current medical approach to chronic illness, limiting the physical symptoms, has its origins in the ancient past and has not changed appreciably over thousands of years. Interestingly the advanced therapies and techniques of modern medicine used today for the treatment of chronic illnesses closely mirror the medical therapies our ancestors used for their afflictions. Although modern medicine would like to present the idea that what is done now is new and unique, the differences between modern and ancient medicine are not as impressive as one might imagine. The greatest differences are the tremendous advances in technology and ready availability of medical care, especially emergency care. Even though our technology today is the stuff that could be pulled from science fiction novels, for many aspects of health care the medical approaches of today and of antiquity are not dramatically different. The reasons are twofold: what worked in the past still works today as the chronic illnesses of today were also the chronic illnesses of the ancient world; and the people of the ancient world were smart and inventive. Archeological records show that the ancient Greeks, Egyptians, and many others suffered from asthma, heart disease, diabetes, infections, bowel issues, and cancer, just as we do today. Even though they may not have known about microorganisms, the immune system, and neurotransmitter molecules, in the ancient world physicians were astute, inquisitive, and resourceful. For the treatment of wounds they fashioned honey and herbal poultices. We know today that honey and many herbs have profound antibacterial, antiviral, and antifungal properties. Indeed in many ancient cultures herbal preparations containing naturally occurring antibiotics were used long before Sir Alexander Fleming received the Nobel Prize in 1928 for discovering penicillin. Using a clay pot and a hollow reed, Egyptian physicians fashioned an effective inhalant therapy for asthma. With the pot upside down on a flat surface a hole was cut in the base. The hollow reed was placed into the hole and specific herbs were burnt under the pot. The asthmatic patient would breathe in the herbal concoction for relief of the asthma. This is very similar to the nebulizer inhalers used today for the treatment of an acute asthmatic episode. There is also evidence of the regular use of surgical tools over five thousand years ago in Egypt and earlier cultures that are almost identical to those used today. This suggests that the types of surgery done today mirror that which was done in the distant past. One specific form of surgery involving the removal of a piece of bone from the skull, trepanation, is especially old. One skull, over nine thousand years old, discovered near Kiev, Russia, has evidence of not only trepanation but also of healing, indicating that the person lived for a significant time after the procedure. Although many archeologists postulate that trepanation was done to "release" evil spirits, there is little evidence to indicate that these cultures believed that evil spirits resided in the skull. An equally likely scenario is that they knew that bleeding in the brain after head trauma is often fatal and that releasing that pressure can be lifesaving. According to Atlanta legend (for those of you who believe that the civilization of Atlantis existed), Atlantean physicians were able to manipulate and modify human and animal DNA by using various frequencies of light and sound. Today we also modify the genetic code in bacteria, plants, and animals. That is how GMO (genetically modified organism) plants and animals are created.

Our ancestors were primitive neither in thought nor in action. It is mystifying to me that we accept the premise that ancient societies were medically primitive and yet had the architectural and engineering prowess, using only bronze chisels, sand ramps, and ropes, to build the something as phenomenal as the pyramids of Giza. The great pyramid alone is composed of 2.5 million stones ranging in size from two to fifteen tons. According to some historians it was built over approximately a twenty-five-year period. That would mean that one stone would have to be placed correctly on the pyramid every 5.2 minutes, 24 hours per day, and 365 days a year for twenty-five years. Even if it took one hundred years to build the Great Pyramid of Giza that would mean a stone must have been cut, transported and laid down every 21 minutes. This is an accomplishment that even with our best technology to date would be impossible. Yet many accept without question that the societies that spawned these ancient engineering wizards were woefully ignorant of illness and medicine. Our ancestors, no doubt, knew more of medicine and illness than we give them credit for, and like the medical approach of today, much of ancient medicine seems to have been focused on the relief of the symptoms of chronic illness. I believe that today we need to do better. Although over the past fifty years the technology of medicine has made exceptional advances in defining the pathology of chronic illness, the treatment mindset remains rooted in medical practices dating back five millennia. Nineteenth-century writer Alphonse Karr summed it up nicely, *"The more things change, the more they are the same."* However today I believe that we have finally reached a turning point. Many people are claiming a more active role in their health-care and I affirm that this is the dawn of the "Age of Healing Miracles."

It is important to understand the limits of traditional and nontraditional medicine so that one's expectations match reality. If success in healing were only based on advertising from medical centers, pharmaceutical and insurance companies, and questionable claims of effectiveness of nontraditional medicine from internet sources, one might presume that miraculous cures for chronic illnesses are happening every day. If these claims were actually true, this book would not need to have been written. Unfortunately, even with our impressive medical technology a reliable cure for any chronic illness is quite rare. For much of the history of humankind the role of medicine was to provide comfort, reduce symptoms, and ease suffering as the patient either lived or died. That emphasis has not changed. Modern medicine concentrates its research, education, and money on those medications and therapies that delay illness-related death, not illuminating what is needed in order to establish a state of health. Physicians prescribe blood-pressure-reducing medications because high blood pressure can lead to death. We want to control the blood sugar in diabetics with medications because elevated blood sugar levels increases the risk of death. Anti-coagulants are used to thin the blood because wandering blood clots may result in a stroke and death. We presume, quite correctly, that if the symptoms of a chronic illness can be managed or reduced we are preventing premature death. Both traditional and nontraditional medicine can be effective at reducing the symptoms of a chronic illness. In this regard they are competing for the same customers. However, preventing premature death is not the same as achieving an acceptable standard of health. Health can be defined as freedom from the medical system itself. Unfortunately, how to secure health-the condition of an organism or one of its parts in which it performs its vital functions normally or properly (Merriam-Webster medical dictionary)-is a distant land foreign to most practitioners of any modern medical arts. For example, in the text book I used while in medical school, Harrison's *Principles of Internal Medicine* (14th edition), there is only one index reference to health, totaling one-and-a-half pages in a 2,500-page textbook with really small print. In those one-and-a-half pages, the main focus was on the cost savings with early diagnosis and pharmaceutical interventions, not on how to establish a state of health. For better or worse, traditional physician training, and much of nontraditional provider training, emphasize naming the illness (the diagnosis) and then recommending whatever medications, surgery, supplements, and therapies will minimize the symptoms (the prescription). These are the metrics by which insurance companies and governmental agencies measure the worth of a physician-how well he/she can diagnose and prescribe within a poorly defined and variable standard of the practice of medicine that has almost nothing to do with establishing a state of health. Now, my brothers and sisters in nontraditional medicine may take umbrage that I feel many are not too far afield from traditional medicine, but if someone needs to constantly take a lot of supplements and herbs or need some form of regular "maintenance" therapy in order to suppress symptoms, they have not achieved a state of health. They have achieved a state of symptom suppression, which is the sin qua non of traditional medicine.

Although both traditional and much of nontraditional medicine wants us to believe that health is the goal, the reality is that these medical systems are designed to delay death through symptom management, not to cure an illness nor establish a state of health (If you don't believe me, use the Google search engine and look up "manage your disease," [2016] at least fifty-three million pages). Despite its numerous inadequacies, modern medicine is to be congratulated for its profound successes. Over the past one hundred years medicine has achieved exceptional success in fulfilling its primary function: to keep people from dying prematurely. However, medical therapy is often the late application of the emergency brake to a car with two flat tires already skidding off a slick road. Since traditional medicine, and to a great extent nontraditional medicine as it is currently practiced, focuses on reducing the symptoms of a chronic illness, I humbly suggest that these approaches to chronic illness have not evolved very far in the past five millennia. From antiquity to the present, the fundamental expectation of medicine is simply to buy time for the innate healing system to restore a state of health. A true physician or healer understands that for both acute and chronic illness, given time and the right tools, individuals heal themselves. Healing takes courage, effort, and time. Only the courageous heal because it takes a level of fearlessness to make that leap of faith, to let go of what is safe and be in that space between the trapeze bars. Indeed those who are healing and who have healed are not only courageous but often are transformed because they are willing to explore the undiscovered territory of self. Actor and author Lindsay Wagner summed it up nicely: *"A lot of people say they want to get out of pain, and I'm sure that's true, but they aren't willing to make healing a high priority. They aren't willing to look inside to see the source of their pain in order to deal with it."* Courage is the engine and the motive force behind all miracles of healing.

The reality that medicine only buys time was strongly impressed upon me when I was a medical student and later a resident (physician in training) at Rush Medical Center in Chicago. Historically physicians in training were called residents because they were so poorly paid (and still are today) that they had to live in the hospital (their residence) because they could not afford to live anywhere else. Medical residencies in the United States

56

vary from between three to seven years. During my residency, Rush Medical Center was one of the first medical centers in the country to attempt bone marrow transplantation for cancer patients. This process involves strong chemotherapy and sometimes radiation therapy to kill the cancer. These high levels of chemotherapy and radiation also kill the bone marrow. Therefore after chemotherapy and radiation therapy the bone marrow must be replaced by bone marrow from a genetically similar donor (allogenic transplant) or by bone marrow removed from the patient before chemotherapy (autologous transplant). Bone marrow transplantation requires that the patient's bone marrow is completely killed before the donor bone marrow can be injected. This leaves the patient without a functional immune system. Between the time the patient's bone marrow is killed and the donor marrow is able to "take root" there is a period where the patient has no defense against bacteria, fungi, parasites, and viruses. During this time patients are kept in strict isolation and large quantities of powerful antibiotic, antifungal and antiviral medications must be used to stem infections. These medications are needed in order to buy time for the new bone marrow to take root. Unfortunately at the time I was a resident the procedure was not very successful. This was not because of the physicians and nurses. They were competent, intelligent and overflowing with compassion. It was simply that the science was not sophisticated enough to enable this procedure to be successful. Many gallant, pioneering patients, despite heroic efforts, died from their infections, not because there weren't robust doses of medications in their system, but because these medications could not buy enough time. With time, experience, and better medications, many patients have been able to be kept alive long enough for the injected bone marrow to take root and begin functioning. It was then that I appreciated the reality that medicine only buys time with the hope that the body will be able to heal itself.

The concept of health is in need of a substantial paradigm shift regarding chronic disease. Humans are not simply physical machines with interchangeable parts. We are composed of a body, mind, and spirit. Each contributes in some manner to the development and maintenance of a chronic illness, and each must have a role in the healing process. Although medicine does a relatively good job at modifying the physical expressions of chronic illnesses, the current medical system-regardless of vacuous advertising by hospitals and medical center conglomerates regarding treating the whole person, body, mind, and spirit-makes meager efforts towards including the mind in any medical plan. Treating the spirit is left to priests, rabbis, and ministers. However, humans are not machines. We are infinitely more complicated with many interacting and complex systems. In order to achieve health, all three aspects of a human need to be healed or repaired: body, mind, and spirit.

The founder of Taoism, Lao Tzu (6th century BCE), is believed to have said, *"If you do not change direction, you may end up where you are heading."* This statement can be interpreted in different ways. It could mean that if stay on your path you will achieve you goal, or it could mean that if you are heading for a disaster you need to change your direction. In the case of chronic illness you are heading for disaster and need to change your direction. A chronic illness cannot be remedied until the body, mind, and spirit are all healed and working in unison. Eliminating just the symptoms of an illness is like cutting the top off a weed. If you do not remove the root, the weed will re-grow. Some traditional physicians and nontraditional healers are knowledgeable enough to know how to revitalize the intrinsic healing system but they, indeed, are a rare breed. Truly the most miraculous phenomenon of this modern era is an increasing desire for self-healing. This idea of self-healing was artfully expressed by the 20th century author and spiritualist Vernon Howard, *"It is a true miracle when a man finally sees himself as his only opposition."*

Chapter 6

Separation of Self – Medicine's Blind Side

I would venture a guess that most people are in agreement with the notion that we are composed of a body, mind, and spirit. It would also be safe to assume that most people would agree that in order to be healthy, the body, mind, and spirit should work together to that end. One cannot exist, cannot be whole if these three components operate independently from each other. However not everyone understands or even believes that the mind and spirit have

> *"The human body is the best picture of the human soul."*
>
> **Ludwig Wittgenstein**

the more important and active roles than the body in ensuring good health. In traditional and much of nontraditional medicine chronic illness is viewed primarily as a physical manifestation, secondarily as a mental circumstance and the role of the spirit is purely a metaphysical footnote.

We can thank Thomas Aquinas (1225-1274 AD) for our current concept of body, mind, and spirit. Aquinas was a Catholic priest and Dominican friar who lived in the last part of the Dark Ages of Europe. He was a brilliant man and one of the most influential philosophers and theologians in the history of the Catholic Church. During the Dark Ages the Catholic Church was arguably the Europe's most dominant political and economic power. Changes in governmental policy as well as scientific and medical thought could not happen without the blessing of the Pope and Catholic Church. Aquinas realized that science (including medicine) was beginning to awaken from its thousand-year sleep. He was worried that that people would increasingly look to science for answers to their questions rather than to religion, especially for health-related problems. For questions such as "Why do I have boils?" religion's response might be simply that God works in mysterious ways. People were beginning to look to medicine and science for better solutions. It was Thomas Aquinas who first divided the human into physical, mental, and spiritual elements. Matters pertaining to the physical nature of a human being were the domain of the sciences (including medicine) while matters of the spirit remained the exclusive domain of religion. The mind was confusing to both science and religion, then and today. Both talk about it but no one really wants to own it. Thus the foundation of modern medicine was born. One critical result of this division of a human into a physical, mental, and spiritual aspect was that any medical discoveries detailing the complex relationship between the body, mind, and spirit and health were ignored or outright censured.

It is easy to understand why Aquinas was able to view body, mind, and spirit as separate. By this time in history Christianity taught that this physical existence is the prelude to an eternity in either heaven or hell. This suggested that we come into this world as a blank slate and when we leave everything is left behind. Now many religions believe that human existence in this world is a one-shot deal. We are here for a time and then leave to go someplace else forever without end, and who am I to say this is not true? However, if we exist in the physical realm only once and for such a short period of time, it becomes difficult to explain why some people have a healthy life and others do not. I have a good friend who eats and drinks whatever he wants, never exercises, takes neither medication nor supplements yet maintains the same 34-inch waist that he had in high school. If a belief is that we are all equal and here only once, well, that is simply unfair. In contrast, other religions such as Hinduism, Buddhism, and Sikhism believe that this physical world is like a classroom. We are repeatedly reincarnated into the physical world to learn specific lesions, and our activities in one lifetime impact subsequent lifetimes. In some lifetimes we may have chronic illnesses and other times we may be quite healthy. Indeed an early Christian sect, the Gnostics, believed that the teachings of Jesus of Nazareth reflected the concept of reincarnation. From my perspective, although raised Catholic, reincarnation is the only rational explanation for the inequities in the world and this concept may be essential for truly understanding the development and as well as healing of any chronic illness.

BODY-MIND-SPIRIT

If we are indeed composed of three separate and yet interacting elements, these elements—the physical body, the mental state and the spirit or soul—have unique responsibilities and functions. When all three elements are working in unison the result is optimal health. Granted, not everyone will agree about the existence of all three states. Indeed, there are those who, in the absence of solid proof, do not believe in the existence of the spirit. Others might argue that Aquinas was wrong. There is no disconnection between the spirit, mind and body. It is all one living organism with its parts vibrating at different frequencies simultaneously. The body vibrates slowest and the spirit vibrates the fastest. There are those who still would argue that the human is even more complex, composed of body, a mind, and multiple levels of energetic "bodies"…ethereal, astral, mental, causal, etc.

Let us assume, for argument sake, that we are a composition of a physical body, a mind that exists in both the physical (brain) an energetic realm (thought), and an eternal, energetic spirit. Let us also assume that the physical body is directly connected to the mind and the mind is directly connected to the spirit. The spirit and the physical body are connected indirectly to each other through the mind since the mind exists in both the physical and energetic worlds. Others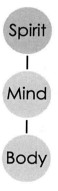

might suggest that the spirit is also directly connected to the body via various glands-pituitary, adrenal, etc. Again for simplicity let us assume that the body, mind, and spirit are connected in the aforementioned, linear fashion.

If one were to list by authority and importance each of the elements that comprise a human, the spirit takes priority. It is actually who or what we really are. The mind and body are simply the extensions of our spirit into the physical world. In this understanding, the spirit is eternal and the mind and body are not. Therefore, the intentions of the spirit have greater value and take priority over the desires of the mind and the needs of the body. The mind directs all of the actions of the body and therefore takes priority over the body. The poor body with no desires of its own gets all of its marching orders from the mind and spirit.

The purpose of each component of a human-the body, the mind, and the spirit-is unique and irreplaceable. The spirit is the primary initiator of life and desire for experience as it is the spirit that manifests itself in the physical plane. One might ask why would something as expansive as the spirit want to come into this physical plane and the answer is straightforward. It wants to experience something in the physical plane that is different from what can be experienced as pure energy, as the spirit. There must be something new to be learned. I spent most of my life in Chicago and its suburbs. There are

> "To enjoy good health, to bring true happiness to one's family, to bring peace to all, one must first discipline and control one's own mind. If a man can control his mind he can find the way to enlightenment, and all wisdom and virtue will naturally come to him."
>
> **Buddha**

certain foods that are unique to this area and one of them is deep-dish pizza. Many, including me, would consider the taste and texture of Chicago style deep-dish pizza a transcendent experience. In those past lives that I can recall I do not believe that Chicago-style deep-dish pizza was ever available. I am certain that one of the reasons my spirit came into this world was to experience, repeatedly, the sublime gustatory adventure known as Chicago-style deep-dish pizza and in this desire my body, mind, and spirit are on the same page.

The spirit needs a way to interpret, categorize, and learn from the various sensations and feelings of the physical world. It needs a mind. The mind is the interface between the physical experience and spiritual understanding of that experience. The mind lives in a hybrid existence in both the physical and energetic worlds. The brain is the physical expression of the mind and it is indeed wondrous. It is densely packed and complex. The adult male human brain is believed to be composed of eighty to hundred billion neurons or nerve cells. A single neuron may connect to a thousand other neurons resulting in trillions of neuron-to-neuron connections. There are also about eighty billion non-neuronal cells that act to support the neuronal cells. The energetic aspect of the mind is that domain through which energy flows, thoughts and ideas are born, and memories, crucial to long-term health, are. According to the famous psychiatrist Sigmund Freud MD, the mind also creates an awareness of itself, the ego. One of the roles of the ego is to interpret and guide the expression of the desires of the spirit into the physical world by directing the actions of the body. However with an awareness of self the ego also develops its own desires and wants to express those desires through the physical body also. Both the spirit and the ego are powerful and when the desires of the ego are dramatically incompatible with the desires of the spirit there can be profound conflict. Since the body cannot serve both the desires of the ego and spirit, there is conflict. To a great degree the physical expression of this conflict is chronic illness. An African proverb perfectly describes this conflict. *"Wapiganapo tembo nyasi huumia"* is translated as "When elephants fight the grass suffers." When the spirit and ego fight, the body suffers.

The spirit longs to expresses itself into the physical world to experience and learn. The physical body experiences the world through its five senses of touch, taste, hearing, smell, and sight. Learning is the treasured result of making bad choices and correcting them. Chronic illness strongly correlates with making bad choices and not correcting them. Recognizing and correcting a bad choice can be a powerful experience, especially if it results in learning and wisdom. Now do not believe for one minute that the spirit on first entry into the physical plane knows anything about the physical plane. It does not. As a result, it makes a lot of mistakes and this is where the concept of reincarnation is important. Over time and reincarnations the spirit makes mistakes and learns and this process can be slow. However it probably does not take many reincarnations for the spirit to learn that trying to pet wild tigers is a poor health choice. On the positive side, petting wild tigers probably reduces the possibility of developing and suffering from a serious chronic illness. The memories of a lifetime of experiences are important in order for the spirit to learn. Even though the brain has only one lifetime, the thoughts and memories are energy. A copy of our ego and memory structure is stored at the eternal level of our existence, our spirit. Some memory of past experiences and decisions come back with us, at least to some degree, at each reincarnation so that we can learn to make better choices. If the phrase "he/she is an old soul" is a familiar one it is because the some concept of reincarnation is embedded deep in our very core. Over many reincarnations the ego eventually learns to align itself with the desires of the spirit, ultimately improving health. Appropriate thoughts and actions afford health and faulty thoughts and actions contribute to chronic illness.

BODY AND MIND

Communication between the mind and body is quite complex. The mind generates a thought. That thought is energy and has a specific vibrational frequency. Positive thoughts have a vibrational frequency that

Mind

|

Body

is probably quite different from the vibrational frequency of negative thought. All thoughts are energy and energy can carry specific information based on the vibrational frequency. The information contained in a thought is gradually transformed from electrical energy to chemical signals through the numerous and complex biochemical pathways of the brain and body. The pattern of energetic thoughts is translated by the physical brain into physical chemicals (neurotransmitters). Neurotransmitters initiate specific and reliable changes in the cells throughout the body. Positive thoughts and their specific vibrational frequencies result in the formation of groups of neurotransmitters that are different from those arising in response to the vibrational frequencies of negative thoughts. In this way the thoughts of the mind are able to be understood and acted upon by the physical body. How this electrical energy is translated into a physical form consistently and with unerring accuracy is still a great unknown. Once these molecules, the physical form of a thought, are received by the individual cells, those cells are compelled to act according to the information. The body cannot override the commands from the mind. If the thoughts are healthy the body will move towards a state of health. If the thoughts are destructive the body is propelled toward illness. The physical body is a perfect soldier. It must carry out ALL the orders without deviation or question, either constructive or destructive, that it receives from the mind.

Thoughts, emotions, desires, and fears do not have a physical existence like a rock or a plant. They are energy and derive their power and

65

authority over the body from the mind. The information that is contained in a thought is brought into the physical world to be made manifest through the human body. Harmonious thoughts, desires, and emotions result in a healthy body. Discordant thoughts and self-destructive desires and emotions contribute to chronic illness. The number of research studies and best-selling books describing the health benefits of meditation, positive thinking and even gratitude are considerable. The health benefits of a simple "thank you" are astounding for both the bestower and the recipient. An act of gratitude makes people happy and happiness is one of the few common lifestyle factors associated with good health among centenarians. In contrast fear, negative thoughts and emotions, and unbridled desires leave a trail of chronic illness and suffering that has been of epidemic throughout recorded history. The downfall of many a kingdom, country, corporation, family, and individual has been the result of negative emotions and desires. Troy, mythical Camelot and Rome all fell, in part, because of undisciplined desires and negative emotions. In modern times, scientific research tells us that high blood pressure, heart disease, obesity, diabetes, cancer, anxiety, depression, etc. are profoundly affected by our thoughts. Our thoughts directly impact our bodies and this is a noteworthy concept. According to the research of Robert Schrauf PhD, Head of the Department of Applied Linguistics at Pennsylvania State University, about fifty percent of our working vocabularies are negative words, thirty percent positive words and twenty percent are neutral words (22). Since words originate in thoughts this means that majority of thoughts are negative and will have a negative impact on the health of the body. In support of these conclusions, I refer to a lecture I attended over two decades ago by Larry Dossey MD on the physical and mental effects of prayer. According to his research, most prayers are pretty negative. Most people are either asking their god(s) to smite someone who does not agree with their specific beliefs, or are praying out of a constant fear that they themselves are going to be smote by their god(s) for deviating from a specific way of life. As an example, when my brother died much of the prayer at his funeral focused on the idea that he was standing at the throne of his God on trial and being judged. All in all, pretty scary negative thoughts and prayers. Many of these prayers asked Jesus Christ to intercede on behalf of my brother to God in order that my brother would be allowed to enter heaven-basically indicating that my brother was somehow unworthy and asking Jesus Christ to become his lawyer. The obvious stereotype was not lost on me. All of the prayers at my brother's funeral were fear-based. I was asked to say a few words and I quoted from the Christian bible a passage found in Corinthians 13:4-8 which is a description of the nature of love. The priest, not a young man, commented that he had never heard this topic mentioned at a funeral. How sad it is that at such an emotionally fragile time, fear rules. Dr. Dossey stated that after publication of his book he received an over-abundance of hate mail, including prayers wishing him ill will, poor health, and even death. He said that the mail simply confirmed his realizations that most prayers are based in negative thoughts and desires. Negative thoughts, even if directed at someone else or some other group of people, also negatively affect the person(s) having those thoughts. Christians in reciting the Lord's Prayer specifically ask to receive in the same quantity and quality the results of their thoughts about their fellow man "...forgive us our trespasses as we forgive those who trespasses against us..." Dossey's book, *Be Careful What You Pray For...You Just Might Get It,* discusses in depth this important concept, especially in regard to prayer. If the most hallowed and structured of prayers are primarily negative, the poorly filtered everyday thoughts probably are dyed an even darker color. Perhaps if our every day thoughts were healthier we would not have the large medical crisis that exists today. There would also be less need for physicians, nurses, hospitals, emergency rooms, medications, therapies, and surgeries. The need for nontraditional medicine practitioners, supplements, and herbs would also diminish.

MIND (EGO) AND SPIRIT

The mind directly affects the body and the body can only respond to the directions from the mind. What about the spirit? This is where it becomes less clear. The research on the spirit's role in chronic illness and health is less certain and opinions abound, including mine.

The connection between mind and spirit is entirely energetic. The mind and spirit communicate primarily through feelings or intuition and to a much lesser extent, thoughts. As an example, intuition is defined by Dictionary.com as a "direct perception of truth, fact, etc., independent of any reasoning process; immediate apprehension." Intuition is a feeling and often a direct communication between the spirit and the mind. Not every thought that pops into the head is intuition. A lot of thoughts may be independent of any reasoning process but have no basis in truth and are certainly not the result of intuition. This is the ego pretending to be more than what it is.

Compelling, deep-seated desires may actually be messages from the spirit guiding the mind and influencing the body to the physical experiences it wants. These desires can be strong to the point of overwhelming. Even as a young child I knew to my very bones that I was going to be a physician. No one in my immediate family was a physician. My mother's family came from England. Her father was a paint and varnish engineer and she became a podiatrist (British term is chiropodist). My father's career led him into the military but during Prohibition his immediate family proudly supplied a substantial amount of the finest Tennessee moonshine to Alfonse Capone's Chicago speakeasies. No physicians are in my

68

immediate family and none of my children subsequently have become physicians. My youngest son toyed with the idea of becoming a physician until he learned that it takes a minimum of eight years of college and three years of residency. Even when I thought that being a professional tennis player was a good idea and it wasn't, I knew deep inside that I was going to be a physician. I earned my Master's degree and PhD before I went to medical school and they opened many opportunities for a career in scientific research. All the same, deep in my "core" I knew that I was destined to be a physician. It was this constant, unremitting message from my spirit that compelled my mind and body to certain actions. All of those actions ultimately led me down the road to becoming a physician. This message was the unrelenting, irresistible force behind my decision to apply to medical school. This same force, my spirit, was the reason I rejected a potentially prestigious career in pulmonary medicine for the lifelong study of integrative medicine which is the combination of the best of traditional and nontraditional medicine. The desires of the spirit always win, and why not? The spirit is who you truly are.

The spirit focuses on the big picture of life and is not involved to any great extent in the mundane, day-to-day activities of life. That is one of the roles of the ego but the ego has its own desires and fears. There are definite experiences the spirit wants or needs to explore and for many people with chronic illnesses it is not the same path upon which the ego wants to travel. The spirit may want to express itself in some creative manner, such as a screenwriter. The ego realizes that there are bills to pay and it enjoys mathematics. 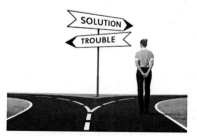 Fearing the uncertainty of employment as a screen writer the ego chooses instead to pursue a career in engineering. These two different paths are seemingly irreconcilable, and therein create the conflict that is at the root of many illnesses. When the spirit wants to go in one direction and the ego, often fearful, wants to go in another, conflict ultimately arises. One might ask why the ego even has fears. Fear is the result of lifetimes of unfortunate experiences usually from making bad choices. If we only enter into the physical plane once, as many believe, we should all have the same fears or the same lack of fears and we don't. Many are afraid of the dark and this may be because of having a few lifetimes cut short by being eaten by something with large, razor-like teeth residing in the dark. The ego remembers and develops a healthy fear of the dark. Some have a seemingly irrational fear of snakes or of drowning– but not everyone. I know of several people who are so panicked at the possibility of public speaking that they needed to be hospitalized. Others cannot get enough of the "bully pulpit." If the spirit wants to move in one direction but the ego is fearful, the physical body cannot travel on two widely divergent paths. It suffers until the ego lets go of its fears and relents to the desires of the spirit. The spirit ALWAYS wins.

Chronic illness is often the result of the spirit and ego moving in different directions. A spirit expresses itself into this world and may want to experience the creative arts like an artist, composer, musician or writer. It may also want to be a physician, engineer or used car salesman. The spirit will push strongly to create this reality. The ego is full of fears and may want to move along a path that leads to financial security and the material comforts that come with it. Eventually the ego and spirit will fight for dominance. A conflict between the spirit and ego creates stress and that stress significantly contributes to the development of chronic illness. The spirit is who you really are. It is the ultimate boss and will not be denied. If necessary, the spirit using a physical illness will stop the ego from moving in a specific direction. I see this played out often in my patients, family, friends, and in me. They are doing what their ego says they should do but not what makes their hearts happy. The internal conflicts and stress over time lead to chronic illness. These conflicts create intense internal stress that can be difficult to treat. It is not unusual for a person with intense internal conflict to present to their healthcare provider with medication-resistant depression and/or anxiety. Others may have chronic insomnia, weight gain, high blood pressure, and type II diabetes. Low self-esteem is common even if the person is highly successful in his/her career and well thought of by others. Often the person is not doing what really stirs their deepest, genuine feelings and moves their hearts. In contrast, they are doing what they believe they are supposed to do and that only feeds the ego.

A middle-aged female sought me out because of her depression and insomnia. She had seen many traditional and nontraditional medicine practitioners without relief. All the medications, psychological therapies, supplements, acupuncture, and even energy-based therapies did not have any lasting effect on her depression and insomnia. Although she was a very successful accountant, it was not the career she really wanted. She wanted a more creative career but her family pushed her towards accounting because it was safe and she could make a good living. She was good at it, had a very comfortable life, a loving husband, and three wonderful children. Given her idyllic life she could not understand her level of depression. With all of her good fortune she felt guilty about being depressed. Eventually the depression and insomnia became so bad that she could no longer work or take care of her family. Multiple extensive and expensive traditional medical evaluations looking for physical reasons of her illness was unrevealing. She was told many times, "Everything looks good," "You should be happy," and "It's all in your head." As a result, she had a bathroom cabinet filled with expensive and ineffective prescription medications. Non-traditional practitioners diagnosed her with adrenal fatigue, systemic candidiasis (a type of fungal infection), low hormone levels, and the non-traditional medicine diagnosis of last resort, toxin overload. She had shopping bags filled with supplements and "detoxification" programs. One energy healer even said the patient was under psychic attack and needed to give her $20,000 in cash (small bills) and an expensive Rolex watch. The energy healer said that she would use the watch to trap the "evil spirits." The energy healer told the patient that after trapping the "evil spirits" she would then destroy the watch ending the psychic attack. I hypothesized that evil spirits must have expensive tastes preferring to be trapped in a Rolex watch rather than a less expensive Timex. When I met the patient I did not believe that a psychic attack was actually happening. I have been the recipient of a psychic attack by something truly evil and it was definitely was not an event that could be resolved with a Rolex watch, even a very expensive one. Fortunately a real, directed psychic attack is quite rare. I would have not been surprised if the "evil spirit"-infested Rolex watch was soon offered on eBay. Even though the patient had a relatively stress-free life I suggested that her spirit and ego were fighting and that the spirit was winning. She was prevented from continuing in the direction preferred by the ego. The spirit ALWAYS wins. The sooner you stop fighting it, the faster you will heal. The patient knew deep down that she wanted a more creative career because her spirit had sent her these messages her whole life. Her fears of financial insecurity compounded by the financial fears of family and friends were stopping her from experiencing a more creative life. Instead she was taking the safer path. However, the spirit will not be denied. Deep inside she knew this was true and it made her depressed and unable to sleep. Part of the healing process included suggesting opportunities for her creatively to express itself. Within a month, the patient moved towards a path that allowed her creativity to express itself without fear or restriction. Her depression improved dramatically and insomnia resolved. She no longer needed her medications. Her spirit and ego had reached an accord and the desires of the spirit were finally being satisfied. She still does some accounting because there are bills to pay but now spends a significant amount of time feeding her creative side.

The faster we realize who and what we are, the faster we can assume complete responsibility for our actions and the faster we can start to heal. At this time in human history, we are rapidly evolving and miracles are everywhere

Chapter 7

The Patient-Driven Transformation of Medicine

The framework upon which the current medical system was built is specifically designed to prevent premature death, and our medical system does this better now than at any time in the long history of man. Because medicine has been so successful in preventing premature death, preventing death has come to be seen as equivalent to creating health. This result has become the driving force for this concept to permeate

> *"If you always do what you have always done, you will always get what you have always got"*
>
> **Anonymous**

every aspect of modern medicine. As a result, medicine has been disinclined to explore new lands, convinced as it is that it is on the right path. Modern medicine is doing what it has always done and we are getting what we have always gotten. The unfortunate result of medicine's success in preventing premature death resulted in a medical system so large that it is incapable of seeing its own limitations. Therefore the stimulus for change must come from the patient. This is evident in the growth of non-traditional medicine and its tacit acceptance by the traditional medical system. This is not the result of mountains of scientific research, but rather because millions of people are recognizing the limitations of medical care and are demanding a change. As the patient population changes and evolves in their understanding of chronic illness, medicine has been forced, to some extent, to evolve in order to stay relevant. It is the patient who drives the medical system, not the other way around. Patients, you and I, are looking for answers to chronic illness, and these answers are rarely found in traditional medicine. That is why nontraditional medicine has become so popular and continues to grow. However, we are not satisfied with either traditional or non-traditional medicine because neither medical system has all the answers. No longer satisfied with the status quo, some people are actively searching for the answers that will lead them to real physical, mental, and spiritual health. People want the whole enchilada and many are willing to do the hard work to get it.

Prior to the early 1900s, the standard of practice of medicine in the United States more closely resembled the lawlessness of the Wild West. There simply were no governing bodies, no standards of practice, and no rules whatsoever. There wasn't even a glimmer of standardization of teaching in any of the medical systems. Anyone-and I mean anyone-could hang a sign over their office and start practicing any kind of medicine, even surgery. The American Medical Association (AMA) was incorporated in 1897 and by 1904 sought to restructure and standardize medical education by creating the Council on Medical Education. The Council on Medical Education recognized the calamity known as medical education and commissioned Abraham Flexner to evaluate all of the medical schools in the U.S. Flexner visited all 155 medical schools in the U.S. and was scathing in his evaluation in all but six medical schools. Johns Hopkins, co-founded by Sir William Osler, was one of six medical schools praised as models of medical education. In 1910, the Flexner report strongly advocated dramatic changes in the educational standards at all medical schools based on the Johns Hopkins model. His recommendations regarding the standardizations of medical education resulted in the closing of many traditional medical schools. Since non-traditional medical schools did not want to follow these recommendations, almost all of them also closed. The wisdom of non-traditional medicine like osteopathy, homeopathy, chiropractic, and naturopathy were almost lost to the pages of American history. Other commonly used nontraditional medical systems like Oriental medicine and Ayurveda (India) were introduced into the United States at a much later date. Some would say that the action of the AMA was an overt power grab designed to eliminate all other competitors and to a large extent this may be true. However, in defense of the actions of the AMA, these changes ushered in a period of unequalled advances in the understanding and treatment of acute disease and the prevention of death. Within a few generations these advances resulted in a doubling of the average American's lifespan. Discoveries in pharmaceuticals and surgical advances were important. Widespread implementation of emergency medical services also contributed. Before all the credit goes to modern medicine, an even greater contributor to the increase in lifespan was the widespread implementation of plumbing along with advances in sanitation. However, a longer lifespan has, in part, played a role in the rise of chronic illnesses of today. Those medical approaches and tools that had proven so successful in treating acute illness and preventing death have failed miserably in treating chronic illness. Traditional and nontraditional medicine need to embrace an expanded vision of chronic illness. They need to be open to the real probability that although chronic illness is expressed in the body, its origins lie in the interactions between the mind and the spirit.

When I was in medical school the emphasis was on the physical expression of illness: the accurate diagnosis of an illness, its patho-physiology, and which medications and therapies reduce the symptoms. Other issues related to health were deemed less important. I have a pretty good memory and can remember only one lecture on nutrition. I can all but guarantee there were no lectures about how to help a patient become healthy. Some of that has changed in the more progressive medical schools. Indeed, Loyola Medical School (Maywood, IL) sends some students to rotate through non-traditional medicine and integrative medicine clinics, including mine. Early in my medical training I was told that ancient medical therapies like acupuncture were at best a placebo response and at worse an outright flim-flam. Since then over 2,000 medical articles and studies published in the American medical literature say otherwise. Herbs were largely effective and potentially dangerous yet over 8,000 medical articles disagree. Bio-energy healing was a fraudulent belief rooted in "primitive" shamanism. Today, there are over 2,000 medical papers on Reiki, a form of bio-energy healing, alone. Chanting and other sound-based therapies are primitive primeval and have no place in "serious" medicine. As published in the medical literature, sound-based therapies can accelerate tissue healing and even modulate how genes are expressed in the DNA. Several years ago a number of the nation's best medical schools recognized that medicine must become more inclusive and formed the Academic Consortium for Integrative Medicine & Health. Their mission is "to advance integrative medicine and health through academic institutions and health systems." Now more than seventy of the top medical schools in North and Central American are members. The "environment" is fertile again for rediscovery of forgotten knowledge. I would venture to say, however, that even with all of the new medical research, as well as the evolution of medical education within these august medical schools, addressing the healing of the mind is rare and healing the spirit is not much more than a philosophical discussion. Medicine is transforming, albeit slowly, not because of a recognized need for a necessary transformation but because you, the patient, are demanding something better and are forcing this transformation. Modern medicine is beginning to recognize the necessity of integrating both the traditional and non-traditional because neither alone will survive. Some medical centers are leading the pack and for others it will be decades before they awaken to this reality. There is now a medical board certification for Integrative Medicine by the American Board of Integrative Medicine (ABOIM) and

American Board of Physician Specialties (ABPS). Even with this medical transformation, recognizing that chronic illness is the result of distress not only within the body but also the mind and spirit will be a long time coming. So it is up to you and me to create the health we all want. This realization is a true miracle in the making.

EVOLUTION OF MEDICAL THERAPY

Today - Treat the Symptoms

The primary focus of both traditional and most non-traditional medicine is merely the relief of physical symptoms. This is the mindset of most in the medical field-physicians, administrators, medical centers, hospital networks, insurance companies, and the government. However if only the symptoms of a chronic illness are relieved, the underlying reason for the illness is unchanged and the underlying illness may get worse. If the root cause of an illness is not corrected, eventually the illness will overwhelm the effectiveness of most treatments. A good example of this can be found in how an autoimmune disease begins. An autoimmune disease is the result of the immune system, the white blood cells, persistently attacking its own body. Although there is a strong genetic component to some autoimmune diseases, an external trigger(s) is often postulated to be necessary for the process to begin. The way an autoimmune disease is usually treated is by suppressing, with strong pharmaceuticals, the ability of the white blood cells to function. This approach destroys the immune system so that it cannot function, hoping that will reduce the symptoms of the autoimmune illness. This approach is only treating the symptoms and not the underlying cause. This is an important concept because if the underlying reason for the disease is unchanged the disease persists and is considered "incurable." Since the root cause has not been addressed, over time, stronger medications with more side effects are often needed to suppress the symptoms.

The Future - Getting to the Root, Changing Destiny

Over the past thirty years, medicine has changed dramatically. Three decades ago the benefits of nontraditional medicine were not seriously considered by traditional medicine. Today it is taught, to some extent, in many medical schools. The medical board certification in the medical subspecialty of integrative medicine (the medical practice of both traditional and nontraditional medicine) is proof of change. The earlier biases against nontraditional medicine continue to erode and patients benefit. For example, in 1998 bio-energy therapy was considered "dead in the water" after publication of the "Rosa Study" in the Journal of American Medical Association and yet today energy-based therapies such as Reiki are common in many prestigious medical centers. Medicine is slowly evolving into a bigger and more complete medical system. The driving force for this evolution is not just scientific discovery but a growing realization by patients that there is more to health then what has been offered in the past. Patients are the prime movers to change in the medical system. They see farther and want to move faster than the traditional medical system is currently able to do. Patients want to get to the root of their chronic illnesses and heal it. They want to be healthy and they want it now.

I treated a patient who had diffuse joint pain, skin rashes, sun sensitivity, and an elevation in blood tests specific for a serious autoimmune disease, systemic lupus erythematosis (SLE). She was initially started on a powerful steroid, prednisone, and her symptoms quickly resolved. Within six months, the symptoms returned and her daily dose of prednisone was increased. The underlying reasons for her illness were many, complex and, in my opinion, strongly related to her mind and spirit. The issues with the mind and spirit were not addressed by either her physicians or by her

80

nontraditional practitioners. Her symptoms worsened. Within a year, the patient was not taking prednisone because it was no longer effective. Over the next decade increasingly stronger medications were needed to suppress the symptoms until there were no stronger medications to be found. The side effects of these medications affected her heart, liver, eyes, and even bone marrow. She was told that there was nothing to be done. She had a strong mind and did not believe that there was nothing and took it upon herself to change her own destiny. In desperation she began to look outside of the box, seeking a greater truth about her illness. Her perception of self was quite negative and at any opportunity she would aggressively belittle and question her actions and decisions. My patient felt that she was not good enough and attacked herself constantly just as her immune system was attacking her own body. In contrast, friends and coworkers felt she was extremely confident, a powerful friend, and very reliable employee and leader. I recommended dramatic changes in her diet, other lifestyle changes and, through energy-based therapies, looking inside her-self for the answers. She followed my recommendations and things began to change. After several years, she passed from this world, quietly in her bed, at the age of ninety-one. She had whittled down the number of medications from seventeen to three and all her symptoms of SLE were gone. She had healed herself and had changed her destiny. Simply miraculous.

Another patient of mine with rheumatoid arthritis, an autoimmune disease, was on a number of powerful medications to limit the progression of the illness. She had been an accountant most of her life because accounting "paid the bills." She was very good at her job but she was overly compulsive about her work and almost everything else. My patient worked long hours and the last time she took a real vacation was measured in years. The rheumatoid arthritis was especially bad in her fingers and it was increasingly difficult for her to use a keyboard and mouse. She also could not sleep because of the pain, and she suffered from constipation over many decades. Her physicians, very competent and highly regarded, had little to offer her except to manage the symptoms as best they could with increasingly strong medications. She hated the way she looked and felt. She was despondent thinking that this hard road she was walking was her destiny. When I saw her, I could envision her as completely healthy. I did not feel she was broken, just out of balance. Without going into all of the details, with changes in diet and select supplements, her bowels returned to normal and her pain improved. Most of the immune system resides in the bowels, and in my experience, healthy bowels and autoimmune diseases rarely co-exist. Earlier in her life, the patient was also quite creative with an emphasis on interior design; however, on her parent's insistence, she gave up what she loved to do in order to have a responsible and safe career in business. After some energy-based therapy sessions, she developed clarity about where her path had gone wrong and began to seek out what she really wanted to do with her life. Most importantly, she forgave herself for deviating from doing those activities that made her "heart" happy. She began to realize that the loss of function of her hands from the rheumatoid arthritis was actually preventing her from continuing on the path of accounting. With this epiphany, she began, without guilt, to do those activities (art and dance) that made her happy. The need for control lessened and her symptoms of rheumatoid arthritis rapidly melted away, especially the pain and swelling in her fingers. Even the blood tests indicating rheumatoid arthritis normalized. Soon she was off her medications. She is still working in business but also is doing what makes her happy in interior design (and making a little bit of money to boot). Miraculously, she was able to rewrite her life story, to change her destiny.

Both of these people realized that the answers they were seeking could not be found by simply reducing the physical expressions of their chronic illnesses. They wanted to be healthy and in order for that to happen they dug deeper within themselves in search for answers. THEY changed their destinies.

Miracles

Chapter 8

How We Actually Heal

One of the great mysteries in medicine is how we are actually able to heal from injury. Traditional physicians and some nontraditional practitioners study in great detail the pathology and physiology of the healing process, from the initial injury to the resultant inflammation to the healing of the injured tissue. We have understood, for a while, much of the process by which a myriad of different cells create many of the critical compounds necessary to promote

> *"Much of your pain is self- chosen. It is the bitter potion by which the physician within you heals your sick self.*
>
> **Kahlil Gibran**

healing and regeneration. It is an integral part of medical education. What we do not know is how this is actually coordinated. Who are the architects and the master builders directing all of these processes, in the correct order and perfect execution, in the right measure and in the right location? Where is the scaffolding that, after damage, new tissue is laid down upon in such precision? Who or what is the intellect that creates with exquisite complexity the discipline of healing out of the seeming chaos of injury and disease? If a house is damaged by a fire (injury), someone has to tear down the damaged portions (inflammation) before rebuilding (restoration) can be undertaken. Each process of rebuilding must proceed in a specific manner and precise timing. Plumbing cannot be done before walls are erected, and wood flooring cannot be laid down before the roof. How is it possible that the cells of a shattered collarbone can come together, almost perfectly, to create the bone anew? At the cellular level this is the equivalent of building a bridge from New York to

London, starting at both locations simultaneously and meeting perfectly in the middle and all without an obvious blueprint. Healing is not a random event. Its consistency across billions of years and innumerable organisms are one of the great and constant miracles of life itself. In humans there is a "road map" for healing and everything involved in the process—body, mind, and spirit—must follow, step by step, this master plan for healing to occur. Chronic illness often results when the mind (ego) and spirit are following different plans and the body cannot serve two masters. So the body and, ultimately, the mind suffer until everyone is on the same page.

Early in my medical career I suspected that not everyone wants to heal. I was wrong. Everyone wants to heal and no one enjoys chronic pain and life altering disability. However there are those who, for a variety of reasons, seem to hold fast to their chronic illnesses and they suffer. A common reason impeding the healing process is that the patient is punishing him/her self for some "unforgivable" sin. The chronic illness is perceived as a way to "pay" for their transgression(s). Miserably, it does not matter how much or how long a person suffers because, in their mind, the debt can never be paid in full. I use to think that many of these faulty thoughts were locked away in the subconscious mind and relatively inaccessible. However at this point in time I believe that most people have some notion about their "unforgivable" sin(s). In these cases the first step in healing is encouraging the patient to recognize and let go of the faulty thoughts that support the "unforgivable" sin. I know this because for a time this was me. Recognition and correction of this faulty thought must happen not only at the mental level but also at the spiritual level. Forgiveness of self at both levels must occur (again, personal experience) for healing to happen. Since the unforgivable sin is a thought its basis in existence is energy. In these instances, bio-energy-based therapies can be an uncommonly effective promoter of this healing process. Medications, supplements, and many of the psychological therapies often fail because their primary place of action is in the physical realm.

Some people, although not wanting to be in pain, do not want to completely heal because, knowingly or unknowingly, they use their illness to manipulate others for their own purposes. With a chronic illness, the extra attention from their spouse, family, and friends may be a motivating factor in maintaining the status quo. Rarely is this for nefarious purposes. It is usually to maintain some feeling of control over their lives. In my experience these types of patients often bounce from physician to physician and healer to healer without any improvement in any symptoms. In their mind their chronic illness is exclusive to them or at least vanishingly rare and will never get better. It is their incurable illness that makes them unique or special and they are right in their belief that their illness is incurable. As long as they hold onto their incurable illness, it cannot and will not be ever be cured. They are the most difficult patients to treat, and healing often spans lifetimes.

Chronic illness can be the catalyst needed for rapid, transformational change of the physical, mental, and spiritual bodies. Transformation is the process that enables us to decipher and understand our particular road map to health. I know of no patient who is so impenetrable that they are not changed in some manner by the experience of chronic illness. I have had a few who really fought change and were pretty darn dense but eventually accepted the transformation process. With positive change, a chronic illness often improves or abates. A transformational change must start with a change in attitude and perception of self. All healing is transformational and fuel improvements in lifestyle such as a better diet, quitting smoking, moderating alcohol consumption, better sleep, increasing exercise, and reducing stress. This transformational change also includes self-forgiveness and putting one's health at or near the top of a priority list. The next step involves an active search for those activities that create a sense of happiness. Amazingly this often involves a needed regression to an almost child-like state of wonder about the world. A person who cannot find anything new or exciting in the physical, mental, and spiritual worlds will not heal in this lifetime. For a number of my patients I recommend that they go to (or back to) college, take courses that are totally foreign to them, and take the courses for no credit. In this manner they can rediscover the wonders of experiencing, without the expectation of achievement, the ever-expanding new and novel aspects of life. In contrast, without engaging in some form of transformational process, chronic illness creates more negative thoughts and feelings as well as physical pain and suffering. The chronic illness only worsens. Moving in either a positive or negative direction is a personal choice. Incapacitating chronic illness is not an inescapable, predetermined eventuality.

Much of the healing of chronic illness is the responsibility of the individual and this healing must originate from within. Tapping into this restorative, internal healing process that we all possess is similar to the process of alchemy. Alchemy is commonly believed to be a quasi-scientific aspect of chemistry with the goal of transforming lead into gold, finding eternal life, and even discovering the mythical universal solvent (a solution that dissolves everything including the container that holds it). On deeper inspection, serious alchemists were not interested in the banal transformation of cheap metals into precious metals. Indeed, alchemy was about a personal transformation from a lower level of existence into a more evolved level of existence and in the process literally healing one-self physically, mentally and spiritually. It is in the understanding of an alchemic transformation of self that we may find the answers to the motive force behind our own health and healing. This alchemic process is the key to health, the transformation from a chronically unhealthy state to a healthy state physically, mentally, and spiritually. In traditional and nontraditional medicine we might say that it is the healthcare provider, physician, nurse, and others who labor on the front lines of clinical medicine who are the alchemic triggers of healing. Others might suggest that it is the researchers, uncovering the truths about how the human body repairs and heals, and discovering new medications and therapies that they are the primary force behind healing. Without their discoveries we would certainly have a markedly limited and ineffective healthcare system. What of the government, pharmaceutical companies, supplement manufacturers, and inventors of life saving medical devices? Certainly they have a vital role in the current medical system and an impact on health. An argument can also be made for the government and funding agencies. Without their support, medical research would simply be a recreation for the wealthy and even mediocre healthcare would be inaccessible for the average person. In nontraditional medicine similar arguments could be made for the chiropractor, massage therapist, acupuncturist, herbalist, and others practicing culturally based medicine. Regardless of the medical system, there are those who directly interact with the patient, those who discover and invent, those who manufacture, and those who give the money needed for everything to happen. Yet, none of them is the alchemic force behind healing and health. You are! You are your own physician and the only one who can, in reality, heal yourself.

Each person is their own personal alchemist and miracle worker, and the only common factor in all healing. All other players are interchangeable. Without exception, each person is the vessel into which all ingredients are blended and mixed in the alchemic mortar, and health is the final expression. This is an actual transformation of the self by the self from the chaotic state of chronic illness to the disciplined state of health. Everyone and everything else involved in this process is simply a tool, a device, a source of information that is used by the true alchemist in this metamorphic process. If a person is ready to change, healing will occur. In stark contrast is a person who is unwilling or does not know that they are able to transform themselves moving new position along the continuum of health. Nothing in the universe, including God, can force this transformation. Healing involves a physical, mental and spiritual transformation although not necessarily in that order. It is in understanding this concept that real, tangible and lasting health can be achieved. In a theosophy magazine, published in 1918, the quote *"When the disciple is ready, the Master will appear"* can be found. It is often believed that this means that when you are ready someone will come into your life to teach you what you need to learn and that is often true. Another interpretation is that for healing, you are both the student and the Master. When you are ready to heal you will discover that you can and will perform miracles. That is the power of our free will and personal responsibility.

Chapter 9

Intention: Fountainhead of All Miracles

Intention is defined as a determination to act in a specific manner with a specific purpose. It is simply a thought with a direction. Everything starts with an intention and intention often precedes great achievements. Most stories about the creation of the universe start with an intentional thought. Depending on the belief system, some all-powerful being decided that it was time for the universe to be brought into existence. There was the intention of creation and that thought created this phenomenal universe. By most accounts an intention may have been the very first thought in the entire universe!

> *"Every action in life, from putting on socks to landing on the moon, begins with an intention."*
>
> **Patrick Massey MD PhD**

STORIES OF CREATION

➢ Hopi Native Americans believe that in the beginning of all things there were only two: Tawa, the Sun God, and Spider Woman (Kokyanwuhti), the Earth Goddess. All above belonged to Tawa, while Spider Woman controlled everything below. There were no humans or animals until they were willed into being by these Two. That was Their intention.

➢ Taoists believe that in the beginning of time there existed only chaos. The elements and gases of the heavens and earth freely mingled and the organizing principle (intention) was dormant. It lay dormant somewhere inside this elemental cosmos awaiting the right moment to begin the transformation. Once this organizing principle (intention) awoke, the universe began.

- In Judaism, as in Christianity, it is believed that the word of God brought everything into being: heaven and earth, mountains and rivers, and every living thing. The word was preceded by an intention.

- The story of the beginning from the Australian Aboriginal people explains that in the beginning only bare land existed. There was no life on Earth—no animals, no plants, no trees, and no humans. Wandjina, the creator, brought the ancestors from within the earth and over the seas, and life began. Again creation began with a thought of intention.

- In the Mayan belief, the Creators, Heart of Sky and six other deities including the Feathered Serpent, wanted to create human beings with hearts and minds who could "keep the days." It was Their intention that brought forth humanity.

- According to Buddhism teaching at the beginning there was absolutely nothing. Brahma the Creator thought, "Let me have a self," and He created the mind. As He moved about, water was generated and the froth on the water solidified to become earth. His luminance became fire. That was His intention.

- The Cherokee creation belief is based in their reverence for the Great Spirit who created the earth for Her children. The Great Spirit who is also called Creator is believed to be omnipotent, omnipresent, and omniscient. The intention of the Great Spirit was to provide a place for Her children to live and thus was formed the earth.

If intention was the source of all creation then the energy involved with an intention can (must?) be overwhelmingly powerful. Without intention nothing happens, literally nothing. Interestingly, traditional medicine recognizes the importance of intention. In medical terminology the word intention is used to describe how an open wound heals. It is literally the intention of the body to heal the wound. If there is no intention to heal, healing does not happen. If a person is resigned to the faulty belief that chronic disease is their destiny and that they have no other options than to carry this burden then the intention to heal never materializes. There might be hope, as in "I hope I get better," but hope is a far cry from intention. Hope depends on chance or the benevolence of others. Intention is an irresistible command that is focused and powerful. Without the intention to heal, chronic illness persists.

When a physician meets a patient it is the physician's intention to do all that is possible to relieve their suffering. That intention is the same for chiropractors, acupuncturists, nurses, physical therapists, massage therapist, psychologists, and everyone in the healing arts. Yet even with all of that forceful intentional energy happening every minute of every day, nothing happens unless the patient creates their own intention to heal; not just relying on the desires and actions of others but doing it themselves. Without a personal intention to heal, no power in the universe can force health on anyone. Intention is the ONLY key that unlocks the power of self-healing and the next step after intention is assuming personal responsibility for the actions needed to fulfill that intention.

This powerful effect of intention is evident in medical research and is known as the placebo response. A placebo response is a perceived or actual improvement of a specific medical condition when a person is given a substance or therapy that should have no effect. For example a person is given a sugar pill for anxiety and believing it to be a real medication, their anxiety improves. The published medical studies debating the true impact of the placebo effect on healing vary. Some research suggests that the placebo effect is small while other studies indicate that, for some chronic illnesses, the placebo response can be quite large. Many medical studies

93

are set up as double-blinded and placebo-controlled. Double blinding means that neither the participants in the study nor those running the study know if a specific participant is receiving the active medication or a sugar pill (placebo) until the study is completed and after the results are tabulated. A placebo is used as a way to gauge the strength of the placebo response, the intention of the participant to heal, when measuring the effectiveness of the active medication. The effectiveness of the active medication is measured by subtracting the results from the placebo from the results of the active medication. This specific study design is considered to be the gold standard of medical research. However the placebo effect can be considerable and large numbers of participants may be needed in order to see any real effect of the test medication. Indeed in some clinical trials the benefits seen in the placebo group can be greater than the benefits of the medication itself! That is the power of intention.

Intention is critical for all aspects of medicine but is especially important in bio-energy based healing. Bio-energy healing is nothing new. It has been part of the human experience probably as long as humans have been on this earth. In its most basic form it is the infusion of energy into or balancing of the energy systems of the body, mind, and spirit. In traditional medicine this concept is certainly foreign; however, every culturally based medical system uses some form of bio-energy-based therapy. Take Oriental medicine as an example. It is a medical system that is completely based on the concept that all illness is the result of imbalances in our bio-energy system. Basically all illnesses are the result of too much energy, too little energy, or the energy is stagnant and not moving. Every therapy used in traditional Oriental medicine including acupuncture, massage, herbs, meditation, joint manipulation (Oriental medicine joint manipulation predates chiropractic by thousands of years), and movement therapy are designed to rebalance the flow of energy. The practice of bio-energy therapy is becoming more common in the United Stated. Reiki, therapeutic touch, healing touch, chakra balancing, color and sound healing, and others are even available at some traditional medical clinics and medical centers. In my office, energy-based therapies have been available to my patients for over twenty years because they work.

Over the past few decades there have been hundreds of published medical studies on bio-energy healing. Some are high quality studies and others are not. Many show improvements over placebo in various measures of pain, fatigue, heart rate variability, sleep, and stress reduction, and improvement in tumors markers for cancer. In contrast some studies show no benefit at all and, unfortunately, none of the studies demonstrate a consistent cure of any chronic illness. Yet there are many cases of patients having miraculous cures of some chronic illnesses after bio-energy therapy. Energy-based therapies need the intention of the patient in order to be effective. Before doing any bio-energy therapy I ask the patient what they want to have happen during the session, i.e., what is their intention. The vast majority but not all patients show significant improvement of their chronic illness symptoms. Some achieve a complete resolution of their illness. If truth be told, very few of my patients receive just energy-based therapy. They also get diet and stress reduction recommendations, supplements, medications when necessary, and lots of encouragement and education.

> *Color and Sound*
> *a bio-energy therapy that re-sets the vibrational frequencies of the energy centers of the body (referred to as chakras) to their original vibrational frequency. Physical and mental trauma, lifestyle, illness and even medications can cause a chakra to vibrate at the wrong frequency increasing the risk of illness.*

The power of intention was strongly demonstrated in one patient who did receive only bio-energy healing from me. She had a miraculous result and was to some extent the impetus for this book. This patient was in her seventies and had lived completely independently on a small farm on the East Coast. After a life-threatening traumatic event, although physically unhurt, emotionally she was devastated. When I first met her, she was accompanied by her daughter because she had completely lost her ability to function independently. Her anxiety had become so overwhelming that she had to move to Illinois and live with her daughter. Medications prescribed by competent physicians had little effect other than make her sleepy. Behavioral therapies were also ineffective, as were all of the supplements recommended by a chiropractor. She seemed lost. When I met her I was amazed by her physical health. She looked like someone twenty years younger. All the medications she was taking were for her new anxiety and depression. She did not seem to be "broken." To my eyes she appeared to be a musical instrument that was dreadfully out of tune. For this reason I recommended that she only needed some bio-energy therapy, specifically Color and Sound therapy. It was her strongest intention to return to her farm and recapture her independent lifestyle. Her intention was so strong that she was willing to try some "New Age, woo-woo stuff" even though she had, in the past, been quite dismissive of such therapies. I recommended that she have three sessions over a one-week time frame. There was substantial improvement after the first two sessions to the point where she drove herself to my office for the third session. At the conclusion of the third session, she sat up, thanked me for the assistance. Interestingly she did not say that I had cured her but that I had assisted her (and she was quite correct). By the end of two weeks she was back on her farm and completely independent. Her intention directed the healing energy to those parts of her body and mind where it was most needed.

I believe that the key to healing is intention and a person's intention has, to my knowledge, never been controlled for in any clinical trial of any medical therapy. It may be that if a clinical trial goes well, it is the intention of the majority of the participants to heal. This often means that even those receiving the placebo drug, supplement, or therapy still exhibit some improvement. In contrast, without focused intention any benefit is limited. There are numerous examples in the traditional and non-traditional medical community where a person must continuously use some medication, supplement, or therapy in order to minimize the symptoms of a chronic illness. In medicine it is rare that a medication or supplement prescribed for a chronic illness is withdrawn because it is no longer needed. Irreversibility of an illness is the definition of a chronic illness, and therefore, by definition, the medication or supplement is needed forever. Indeed, often it is the intention of the physician or non-traditional practitioner that the patient takes the medication or supplement forever. As a result, the intention of the patient is to take the medication or supplement as directed because they want to experience the symptoms of the chronic illness. So ingrained is this concept that I do not recall the topic of reversibility of a chronic illness ever being discussed in medical school or during medical residency. Along the same vein, in nontraditional medicine chiropractic manipulation, and massage therapy is often employed as a form of maintenance therapy. Although a person may feel better after manipulation or massage, the effects do not last, and over time, the person may actually become just as dependent on these therapies as someone taking a medication for high blood pressure. In the absence of a specific intention to heal, many are content to let others manage their chronic illness if it allows them some degree of normal functioning. The same is true for bio-energy therapies. Although millions of people have experienced some form of bio-energy healing, including prayer, and feel better, few are completely cured. Even when treated by incredibly gifted energy healers, real cures are rare. I have been treated by, I believe, some

97

of the best in the world and have had some fantastic experiences. I always felt better after each session. Yet it was not until my focus, my intention to heal changed that my own healing actually began. Those I have treated and who experienced cures have realized, as I did, that they needed to do the actual work. It is their intention to heal themselves. Intention creates miracles.

Chapter 10

How Do I Start To Heal?

After intention, the next most important step for healing is personal choice and the wondrous transformation of self that happens in conjunction with it. This transformation is not easy. Remember that we humans are many-layered beings composed of at least a body, mind and soul. Transformation can be complicated. It can take time. Change is difficult and healing is all about change-changes in the physical, mental, and spiritual

> *"When it becomes more difficult to suffer than to change...you will change."*
>
> **Robert Anthony**

bodies. If change were easy everyone would be doing it. We resist change because it is unfamiliar and most of us do not enjoy exploring unknown. Unfortunately some may consider the suffering of chronic illness preferable to the transformation necessary to heal. Change, however, is the only constant in the universe. Nothing ever remains the same. Eventually the pain of a chronic illness will become strong enough to compel change. For many this can take lifetimes. Those who are tired of suffering are transforming themselves now. Change means entrance to undiscovered territory, and the sooner we explore this great unknown, the sooner we heal. As the incredible comedian George Carlin once said, *"The status quo sucks."*

There is no "one size fits all" in healing because we are all different and are at different stages of self-awareness. For someone who is aware of self, tired of illness, and open to change (the latter being the key), a single word or phrase can result in almost instantaneous healing. In the Christian bible, Jesus of Nazareth healed people with only a few spoken words. It may be that Jesus of Nazareth must have chosen the recipients of healing carefully because for what records there are, he healed very few. It is my impression that just those who were finally open to change, i.e., had the intention, were able to be healed.

The initial step in healing does not happen in the body. It begins in the mind, that part of us that exists in both the physical and energetic worlds. A person needs to recognize that there is a persistent physical problem and that whatever medical therapy they are doing-be it traditional, nontraditional or a combination of both-it is not enough. This initial step is the birth parent of the second part of the process, which is to make changes in lifestyle and look beyond the diagnosis of traditional and nontraditional medicine for answers. The following suggestions should not be taken as individual medical advice but as a guide for further exploration of your unique healing journey. I wish you extraordinary success.

The first step is to recognize that you are the reason for your chronic illness. This is not meant as a condemnation or to elicit guilt. It is simply reality. Most chronic illnesses, excluding the rare genetic illness, are the result of lifestyle and, as an adult, ultimately are your responsibility (knowingly or unknowingly). Accepting responsibility for a chronic illness is a monumental step in healing. The next step is to establish a powerful intention to heal. As I explained earlier, nothing happens without intention. The effect of the intention is a direct result of the level of energy put into it. In the case of healing it needs to be reinforced almost daily. An example of an intention is "It is my intention to use all of my abilities, physical, mental, and spiritual, to understand and heal my (insert your specific chronic illness) now." The energy and effect of intentions are directly related to the energy put into them. There is so much in life demanding a person's attention and can dilute the energy of a healing intention. I believe that a successful healing intention must be handwritten and spoken out loud with commanding authority almost daily. Printing them onto paper and hanging them on the wall will not imbue them with any real power. Successful people literally live their intentions every day, not just hang them on the wall in an expensive frame.

HEAL THE BODY (easiest step)

I.   Diet.

"*Let food be thy medicine and medicine be thy food*" (Hippocrates). Nowhere in the long history of man have people eaten the way we eat today in the United States. A diet high in bad fats, starch, poor protein quality, limited amounts of fruits and vegetables, junk food galore and individual portions so large that they could feed a family of four are the norm and a perfect prescription for chronic illness. I am a big fan of the Mediterranean diet as advocated by Andrew Weil MD as are most physicians and health care practitioners who have completed his groundbreaking Program in Integrative Medicine at the University of Arizona. This particular dietary approach has the most medical research and the outcomes are very positive for a variety of chronic illnesses especially irritable bowel disease, autoimmune disease, obesity, high blood pressure, and diabetes. Other dietary methods may also be helpful including Weight Watchers, South Beach, and various versions of the Paleolithic diet. Vegetable-based diets are also very healthy, but a strict vegetarian approach does not suit all people. A vegan approach is prone to serious nutritional insufficiencies. Even the Dali Lama is not a strict vegan. To me the bottom line is to dramatically limit starches like bread, rice, pasta, and potato. Be aware that additional starch is often added to gluten-free foods to make them palatable. I also recommend greatly limiting soda and eliminating sugar-free anything unless it contains stevia. I am not an advocate for the current recommendations for the consumption of cow's milk. They are excessive and in my opinion may contribute to a number of chronic illnesses. Cow's milk contains at least sixty hormones in quantities that will affect long term health, and bovine milk protein is a strong food allergen. There is a need to increase our intake of organic fresh fruits and vegetables, soups, and lean, organic, non-processed meats. Without a long discussion on the advantages of organic food, take me at my word that organic is better. Minimize the intake of nitrite-containing foods like hot dogs, bacon, sausages, and processed meats, especially if cooked at high temperatures. Nitrites are added to meats as a preservative and coloring agent. Cooking these foods at high temperatures transforms the nitrites in these foods into nitrosamines. Nitrosamines are known carcinogens. Nuts and seeds are very healthy in moderation. Finally, portion control is very important. Eating too much of anything is *unhealthy*. There is increasing medical research on the benefits of fasting. There is not enough good research for me to make specific recommendations, but fasting seems to part of many religious traditions such as Catholicism (Lent), Islam (Ramadan) and Judaism (Yom Kippur). Buddhist monks make fasting a part of their regular routine.

II.   Sleep

Most Americans do not get enough sleep. I have a number of patients who have boasted that they can get by on four or five hours of sleep per day. My response is usually, "Not for much longer." Humans need between seven and eight hours of sleep per night. The best hours for sleep seem to be between 10pm and 2am. After 2am, the body begins to wake up. It is during sleep that the physical body heals and <u>there is no substitute</u>. Sleep deprivation either by choice or job, greatly increases the risk of many chronic illnesses including heart disease, diabetes, obesity, autoimmune diseases, and Alzheimer's disease. Robust medical research has demonstrated that those who work second and third shifts develop altered sleep patterns and have reduced levels of "healing" molecules called endorphins. Consistently inadequate endorphin levels increase the risk of the chronic illnesses list above. Other medical systems also realize the importance of sleep. In traditional Oriental medicine the body is kept in balance by the interplay of two balancing energies, yang and yin. Yang energy is described a masculine, active, hot, bright, and dry. Yin energy is described as feminine, dark, unmoving, cool, and damp. One form of energy is not superior to the other and both are needed for health. Sleep is considered yin. Yin energy is essential for good health because healing happens only during yin. Some believe that during sleep we leave our bodies and travel to other dimensions. We are still connected to our bodies but our consciousness travels outside our bodies. During this time, angels are then able to enter the physical body and initiate and promote various healing processes. Whether it is endorphins, yin energy, or the efforts of angels, proper sleep is crucial to healing and health.

III.   Exercise

It almost goes without saying that exercise is good for everybody and that Americans certainly need to exercise more. In stark contrast to when I was a youngster, lo those many years ago, today less than thirty percent of children exercise on a daily basis (23). Not unexpectedly, fewer than one in twenty adults exercise thirty minutes per day (24) and eight out of ten Americans, both adults and adolescents, do not get enough physical exercise on a regular basis (25).

Across the board almost all chronic illness is made better with physical movement sometimes to the point of healing. The type of physical activity is less important than doing something on a regular basis. However if the exercise is only high impact and tremendously vigorous then it is pretty unbalanced. Unbalanced exercise exerts uneven stress on the body and increases the risk of injury. This may be a compelling reason why professional athletes in football, basketball, gymnastics, and track and field (especially sprints) have a high incidence of significant to career-ending injuries. An active person also needs physical activity that is relaxing (even just relaxed stretching) and should do it in equal measure to more vigorous exercise. I realize that gymnasts stretch and are very flexible but that level of physical strain on a young, developing body often damages tissues and that damage can last a lifetime. In contrast to competitive activities, some exercise like tai chi and yoga can benefit both the body and the mind and perhaps even touch the spirit. Tai chi is often described as moving meditation. Dance also has the ability to not only impact the physical but can free the mind to connect with spirit. The Sufi Muslims will twirl repetitively and for great lengths of time as a way to reach spiritual enlightenment. Experiencing a reality beyond this physical plane may be the real reason why people, across the world and time, love to dance. It has been my experience that the spirit loves music and everything associated with music, including dance. All of the various recommendations for length and intensity of physical activity as well as the cardiac response of a specific exercise program are less important than simply doing something on a regular basis and having fun.

IV. Stress Reduction

No one can handle chronic stress. That is one the great fairytales of the 20th and 21st centuries. Chronic stress is ruthless and cruel. It is a major contributor to ALL chronic illness. It damages all the organ systems and increases the risk of all diseases, including cancer and Alzheimer's disease. It injures the body, damages the mind, and, ultimately, extinguishes that form of essential communication, the light between the spirit and mind. Unrelenting stress results in chronically elevated levels of cortisol, an anti-stress hormone. Consistently elevated levels of cortisol are quite toxic to brain cells and other tissues. This may be one reason why many who are under chronic stress complain of difficulties with memory and cognition. Their brains are literally dying.

Reducing chronic stress must begin with specific lifestyle changes. Toxic employment contributes substantially to chronic stress. If you work in a toxic environment, literally and figuratively, do not be afraid to migrate to greener pastures. I moved from a financially rewarding career in traditional medicine to a career in integrative medicine. I do not make as much money but I have time to stop and smell the roses. My wife and I have been able to afford a nice home, reasonably priced cars, regular vacations, and college for our four children. Even late in my career, I cannot fathom retiring because I love what I do and, unlike much of medicine today, my work is not toxic. Although initially unsettling, a career in integrative medicine was the best career decision and healthy lifestyle choice I ever made. It saved me from the unrelenting stress that is the sine qua non of my physician brothers and sisters.

Interactions with other people are often a source of extreme stress. The most direct and simplest solution is to eliminate toxic relationships. This can be hard because some of these relationships may be with family members. Stressful relationships are a significant source of chronic stress. Ideally, a person should become the "bigger" person and rise above the stress caused by a toxic relationship. However that kind of growth takes time, maybe even lifetimes, and for those in the midst of a stressful relationship, time is not on their side. Remember, you can love someone and not like how they act. You also do not have to subject yourself to someone else's actions unless you want to do so. It is a matter of choice and personal responsibility.

The effects of stress are minimized by having fun. Fun feeds the inner child in all of us and the inner child is very powerful. It can and does counteract the effects of stress. I often ask my stressed patients, "When as the last time you had real and lasting fun?" Often there is a long silence and facial expressions of sadness as the patients realize that real fun has been absent in their lives for many years. Some have to go all the way back into their youth to remember a time when they had fun. Life was not meant to be seventy or eighty years of work and pain followed by some vague, promised reward in the afterlife. Life is meant to be enjoyed. At times there will be some work and personal development but the regular enjoyment of life itself is crucial for health and healing. You can work and accomplish goals and still enjoy it. Most of my patients are gridlocked in the responsibility of life and have lost their childlike wonder. Whenever I go to Disneyworld I wear a set of Mickey Mouse ears and allow myself to act silly and childlike much to the amusement of my children and probably mild embarrassment of my wife. My favorite ride in the whole park is "It's a Small World." The music makes me happy, feeds my inner child, and it is fun!

On a regular basis, spend some time alone with yourself and I mean completely alone. By adulthood we define ourselves by what we do, where we live, and the people around us. We often lose that most important of connections, the one to ourselves. That loss increases stress because that is the connection to our spirit. Without a connection to our spirit it is commonplace to feel lost, disconnected, and truly alone even when in a crowd of people. There are many examples of people who during a time of crisis isolate themselves from the outside world in order to "find themselves." If you take time on a regular basis to be alone with yourself you will not be lost and down the road not have to isolate yourself in order to "find" yourself. A prime example of this phenomenon is the mid-life crisis. A person, in later middle age, may abandon what they have and who they have known, usually because they lost themselves in that specific lifestyle. They then move in a radically different direction often regressing to an earlier time when they felt more connected with themselves. All they were really trying to do is to reconnect with their spirit

HEAL THE MIND

Since the mind exists in both the physical and energetic realms, both need to be addressed in order for healing to occur. The most critical step in healing of the mind is to accept responsibility for the chronic illness. In most cultures once you reach the ripe old age of twenty-one you are an adult. At that point in time you can recognize that the actions of others, at an earlier time in your life, may have had an effect on you and your health; however, upon reaching adulthood, everything you do, what you think and do not think, are totally your responsibility. You can no longer blame your parents, family, friends, or even circumstances for your chronic illness. Without being blind or unsympathetic to the health effects serious traumatic events early in one's life, one can insist that as an adult it is your responsibility to seek out those people, methods, and therapies that can help you heal if you choose to do so. The exceptions to this are those with such serious illnesses that they are either physically or psychologically unable to seek help. They must depend to a great degree on the benevolence of others for help.

I.   Healing the Physical Mind

I consider the physical mind to be defined only by its physical parameters, commonly called the brain. The brain is similar to a muscle. If you do not use it, it deteriorates. If you exercise the brain in the right manner it grows stronger. Most people stop learning new things, seeking novel experiences, and expanding their reality by the age of thirty. Lifestyle may play a role since it obviously becomes harder to explore new horizons because of work, careers, family, and ultimately fatigue. Many people get set in their daily routines, and routine is the adversary of learning and growing. New experiences and challenging ideas actually strengthen the brain. Each nerve in our brain is connected to many other nerves. By some estimates each nerve cell in the brain is connected to 10,000 other nerve cells and there are about 100 billion nerves so there are potentially 1,000,000,000,000,000 (one quintillion) connections. The more connections between brain cells, the stronger the brain becomes. New experiences and novel ideas increase the number of new connections making the brain stronger, faster, and more intelligent. A longstanding routine lessens the opportunity for new brain-cell to brain-cell connections. Over time the brain becomes weaker. So to heal the physical mind a person must get out of their comfort zone and have new experiences, lots of them. Mark Twain once said *"Travel (new experiences) is fatal to prejudice, bigotry, and narrow-mindedness, and many of our people need it sorely on these accounts. Broad, wholesome, charitable views of men and things cannot be acquired by vegetating in one little corner of the earth all one's lifetime."* I would say that new experiences are the essential fertile ground upon which a healthy brain is cultivated.

New experiences raise the levels of many neurotransmitters especially those that are commonly associated with reversing the symptoms of depression, anxiety, and insomnia, such as dopamine, serotonin, and gamma-aminobutyric acid (GABA). Exercising the brain with new experiences also strongly stimulates the production of endorphins commonly classified as mood-elevating hormones. This is why vacations are so important for stress reduction and mental health. Astute executives know this and make sure their employees take all of their vacation. It spawns more efficiency and creativity in their employees. New experiences create the desire for more new experiences. This establishes the environment for a life-long strong mind. Go back to college. Take a class you never would have taken in the past. Take it for "no grade" so there can be no expectation of achievement. Just enjoy the experience. Share the experience with friends and family. Then, go do it again!

II. Healing the Energetic Mind

The energetic mind is directly connected to the physical mind but is not the physical mind. In science we still do not know how thoughts form and where they are stored or exactly where the personality is located. Where inside the physical brain is the home of that feeling of uniqueness felt by every living person? A few researchers and philosophers have ever searched for the essence of our individual uniqueness and have named it the "ego." The ego determines to a great extent the quality and quantity of our everyday thoughts and ideas and what we do in our daily lives. Even though the energetic mind is connected to the energetic spirit the inclination of the ego and the desires of the spirit rarely point in the same direction on a compass. It is this disparity that contributes to illness and must be corrected in order for healing to occur.

Healing the energetic mind requires that the ego recognize that is not alone and, more importantly, that it is not in charge. For strong egos this can be very hard and they will resist all attempts at change and transformation. It can be hard for many to realize that there is more to this world than what can be seen or felt. There are worlds beyond worlds both inside and out. Meditation, prayer, and mindfulness are effective ways to train the ego to accept the wisdom and direction of the spirit. Often using these techniques effectively can take a great deal of time and require a level of discipline. In addition, in technologically advanced societies the constant use of technology stimulates the logical thinking part of the brain and feeds the ego. Creative thoughts and feelings are habitually suppressed. The spirit communicates with the mind primarily through feelings and sudden bursts of creative discovery that defy linear thought. Logic is a linear process and feelings do not follow logic. Therefore communication between the mind and the spirit is difficult if feelings are not regularly nurtured. Without regularly experiencing feelings the logical part of the mind does not have a reference point in order to learn from the older and wiser energetic spirit. It can take time for a person, often in isolation, to feel the subtle flow of their own energy and quiet guidance of their spirit. For many a faster way is to experience some form of bio-energy healing. It creates a reference point for the logical mind. I once gave a lecture on alternative medicine to a large group of cardiologists, a pretty conservative, left-brained group indeed. When I began to describe the medical research on bio-energy healing I realized I lost almost the entire audience. I lost them not because the lecture was boring. I give bodacious lectures. They had lost interest because they had never felt the movement of bio-energy. They literally did not have a point of reference for their logical minds. I stopped the lecture and had them do a simple exercise to feel energy and most felt something. After the lecture one of the cardiologists came up to me and said that he still was unsure about the "whole energy thing," but now he had some idea what energy felt like. He had changed his point of view because now he had a point of reference that his logical mind could accept. For many people, experiencing energy-based therapies changes their point of reference from being ego-based to touching their spiritual self. It feels wonderful and can happen fast. In my experience the benefits are most impactful when energy healing is followed by various meditation techniques.

Although I have experienced a number of different meditation techniques, most of them required time and a certain level of discipline before any tangible benefits were revealed. I do have wonderful experiences in meditation, seeing the

> **Inner Sanctuary**
> a meditation technique the establishes a constant and reliable sacred space to rapidly and directly receive answers to questions, release negative thoughts and feelings, restore balance and vitality, manifest creative ideas, and strengthen sense of purpose.

111

unseen and traveling to places not on the usual tour maps. However, I rarely received any direct answers to my questions. One specific technique that I teach some of my patients, Inner Sanctuary meditation, I learned at Delphi University in McCaysville, GA. This specific meditation technique is simple and quickly puts you in direct contact with your spirit where you can get direct answers to questions. Any meditation technique such as qigong, yoga meditation, mindfulness, or progressive relaxation can be beneficial. Like all meditation you need to practice Inner Sanctuary meditation but it is straightforward and the benefits can be rapidly realized.

HEAL THE ETERNAL SPIRIT

The spirit is who we were at the beginning, who we are now, and who we will be in the future. Along the way the spirit accumulates a lot of experiences and memories. These past experiences and memories can help in our current and future lives, but others are simply excess baggage. They may have been beneficial at some point in time but, like clothes that are outdated or too small, they no longer fit our needs. Sometimes we do not want to jettison some of the excess baggage. We are attached to it and feel that we might need it in the future and so we hold onto it. This leftover baggage can be perceived as faulty thoughts. Faulty thoughts affect how we view our lives, relationships, and everything else. They can be destructive and impede the healing process. Racism is an example of a strong faulty thought that exerts its negative effects on everything and everybody. Self-loathing or feelings of inadequacy are powerful faulty thoughts that brings healing and growth to a screeching halt. We all have an abundance of faulty thoughts and they send the wrong messages to the mind and body. The body must act on all thoughts especially those with a substantial energetic force. Powerful faulty thoughts create stress and as discussed earlier, unrelenting stress is the harbinger to chronic illness.

Fortunately there are solutions! Thoughts, faulty or otherwise, require a constant input of energy to exist. If the energy is removed from a light bulb (an LED in these modern times) the radiant glow quickly stops. It is the same for thoughts. If no energy is put into the thought, the thought ceases to exist. In this activity the ego is crucial for the healing of the spirit. The ego determines which thoughts get energy and each person has complete control over this process. A faulty thought can be transformed into a positive thought or it can be removed. Either process accelerates the healing of the spirit by breaking those chains that bind us even if it is only one link at a time. In the story *A Christmas Carol,* author Charles Dickens describes the spirit of Jacob Marley, Ebenezer Scrooge's partner, as being weighed down with chains, "cash-boxes, keys, padlocks, ledgers, deeds, and heavy purses wrought in steel." Marley's spirit was being crushed down by the weight of its own faulty thoughts. Yet, in reality, Marley possessed the power to transform his chains into something beneficial.

Transformation of any faulty thought takes time, sometimes lifetimes. Removing faulty thoughts can be very rapid process but can require some work to make sure another faulty thought does not take its place. Getting rid of one dictator does not mean another will not take its place. Removing faulty thoughts without learning the reason for the faulty thought rarely results in permanent change. Ideally you want to both understand the origin of the faulty thought and then remove it. This is a process of transformation similar to that sought by alchemists mentioned earlier. A person has to seek change in order for change to happen. There are many ways to self examine and heal the spirit, far too many for the pages of this book. I have seen great success with a specific transformational therapy called "RoHun ^{TM}." It is not easy nor for the faint of heart, but if you are tired of suffering, this can be a very effective therapy. Other energy healing therapies, some of which I personally do, are also effective. However not all energy therapies involve the needed transformation of one's self required for lasting healing. As explained earlier, passive healing therapies that just add energy without a specific intention can feel terrific but rarely yield lasting results. Just adding energy to the system can also strengthen faulty thoughts, making the illness worse. The bottom line is that recognizing and releasing (or transforming) faulty thoughts heals and lightens the spirit making communication between the mind and body easier.

Meditation, prayer, self-assessment, and many other similar therapies can be used to heal the spirit. In my experience, as powerful meditation and prayer can be, without the specific goal of understanding the basis of a chronic illness the benefits of meditation and prayer are limited. Meditation should have a specific and focused goal; otherwise it is only a relaxing interlude. A relaxing interlude is nice but it will take a long time for it to change anything. This may be one reason why results from medical research studies on meditation are so variable. Sometimes it is effective and sometimes not. Prayer should also be focused on not just receiving some blessing or forgiveness of sins but on understanding why you feel the way you feel and what you can do to correct it. Prayer also should be accompanied by a quiet time to receive the answers. If you are always talking you cannot hear the answers. The answers most often come as feelings rather than thoughts. If you are receiving thoughts rather than feelings it usually means that you are simply talking to your ego. If praying for health is not accompanied by a desire for understanding and for the strength to do what is necessary to succeed it is only words. God, the Great Spirit, or the universe is not punishing you with a chronic illness. You are! The Higher Powers, like college professors, offer guidance and support during your learning process but do not expect the

Higher Powers to do the work for you. How will you ever develop wisdom if someone does the all the work for you? In the New Testament of the Bible, Jesus of Nazareth did not say to the crippled man at the pool of Bethesda "here, let me carry you and your stuff." He said "Rise, take up your bed and walk."

In the realm of healing of the spirit there are many therapies that offer insight into illness and guidance about healing. They all have advantages and limitations. Remember, they are tools and you still have to do the work.

Bio-energy-based therapy: This process can be a rapid way to experience the many realities beyond the five senses. That is not a "new age, woo-woo" claim. Our five senses are limited to a very narrow energy spectrum. Humans cannot see in the range of infrared or ultraviolet or hear sounds above 20 kHz. Experiencing realities beyond what we normally experience opens the communication pathways to the spirit. This fuels a desire for greater understanding of the roots of chronic illness and healing is accelerated. Color and sound, reiki, Light Energization^{TM}, therapeutic touch, Rohun^{TM}, qigong, and innumerable therapies without names done by those who are proficient in bio-energy therapeutics are some of the many gateways opening communication between you and your spirit.

Past-life regression: Done with the right intention, a past-life regression can offer insight as an inciting initial event in a past life resulting in the faulty thought(s) impacting a chronic illness today. It is not the cure. It is a source of information that can be applied in the present lifetime.

Crystal healing: I like crystals. I like the way they look. I like the way I feel when I hold them and I use them in some of my energy healing therapies. To put them in perspective, crystals are tools. They are not magic. Their consistent and specific vibrational frequencies can help to re-establish and balance a person's various vibrational frequencies that are important for healing. In the right manner crystals can be used as tool to weaken the energy of faulty thoughts, thus accelerating the healing process. They can help a person to remember what health feels like. However it is up to the person to do what is necessary to maintain those healthy vibrational frequencies. Despite new age claims about crystals, lasting healing cannot be done by crystals alone. It is not their responsibility and you must be the driving force for change.

Music and chanting: Everything in the universe vibrates-EVERYTHING. This may be interpreted that everything in the universe sings. Music is a powerful and primal healing energy. As with crystals, if a person is a passive recipient, is only listening, the benefits of music are modest at best. In contrast there can be lasting, positive benefits for individuals if they are regularly singing or chanting. They are creating their own vibrational frequencies that are acting upon themselves. Like crystals, the right frequencies of music can diminish the power of faulty thoughts. That is, to a great extent, why people like to sing even if only in the shower. Music balances and enhances a person's healthy vibrational frequencies and music is an integral part of every culture in the world.

Energy chambers, singing bowls, salt caves, qi generators: These are devices that generate specific frequencies of energy that claim to be associated with healing. Specific vibrations of energy

116

may be associated with healing and may stimulate the intrinsic healing process. In traditional physical therapy the same theory is applied when ultrasound and electro-stimulators are used. They generate vibrational frequencies that stimulate healing of the physical body. These eclectic tools may be beneficial in the short term but again, the person has to do those other activities going forward that solidify the healing process. In the case of physical therapy you have to do your exercises in order to heal. No one and nothing can do it for you despite any advertising claim.

Many of the people I treat are chronically ill and need to heal at the physical, mental, and spiritual levels. I suggest that healing begins at all levels at the same time. The body, mind, and spirit are all connected and work together so healing therapies aimed at the all three, the body, mind, and spirit, work synergistically and often result in a rapid resolution of chronic illness, restoration of health, and a new found zest for all that life has to offer. With all of its problems, the world is exciting. With good health you can appreciate all of the wondrous experiences designed to delight and teach us. It would be truthful to say that the miracles we are all looking for can and are being discovered right now, everywhere.

Miracles

Chapter 11

My Story

This is by far the least important chapter in this book but many have asked me, "How did you start doing this kind of medicine?" Basically it was the combination of good fortune, curiosity, persistence and I listened to my spirit. As a result of a series of unusual events at an early age I recognized that the world is much more complex than we what we usually perceive. Like Einstein, I am passionately curious about many things

> "I have no special talent. I am only passionately curious."
>
> **Albert Einstein**

and have enthusiastically and without any apology explored that which many of my contemporaries would consider unusual.

I was born on a military base in the town of Fontainebleau, France, a small suburb outside of Paris. My father was a technical sergeant in the United States Air Force. A technical sergeant is a non-commissioned officer position between a staff sergeant and master sergeant. He was stationed there with my mother. Later he was stationed to another military base near the small town of Sulfur, Oklahoma. We lived in Sulfur for several years and my sister was born there. It was there that I had my first of many experiences showing me that the world was more complex than what we usually perceive.

Even though I was born robust lad I had a severe heart defect and as a result I was not the healthiest of children. If not for fantastic advances in heart surgery it is unlikely that I would have seen my eighteenth birthday. Often I needed to stay indoors and could not play with the other children. I spent a lot of time alone and it was during an afternoon nap that I had the first of two childhood "out of body" experiences.

In my first experience I began to float-not fall-down a long tunnel. Floating beside me were my toys, teddy bears and little wooden rocking chair. I was floating down faster than my possessions as if I was leaving them behind. At the bottom of the tunnel there was a very bright light. I felt no fear floating down as if gently drawn toward the light. It was a very pleasant experience. Then I suddenly awoke in my bed and told no one of the experience. Sometime later-I am not sure if it was days, weeks or months-the same experience happened again during another afternoon nap. Only this time, I reached the end of the tunnel and I experienced what was on the "other side" of the white light. When I awoke my mother was holding me and crying. At that time I did not understand why, but later in my life my mother told me that she thought I had died. Again, I told no one what I had experienced but kept it close to my heart because what I had learned from being on the other side it was very important to me (and still is). What I saw and why I came back from the other side, either from my mother's love or from some other factor(s), is a story for another time. Maybe it will be the topic of another book. Since I was too young to read about near-death experiences and the only show for children on television was Howdy Doody (Google it) my experiences cannot be dismissed as a figment of the fertile imagination of a child. I suspect that many people have had "near death" or "out-of body" experiences but are afraid to say anything because "experts," without a point of reference themselves, have dismissed such events as fantasy or outright lies. They often insist that there is no scientific evidence for such

120

an experience and therefore it is not possible. In reality there is more evidence supporting "out of body" experiences than refuting it. At one point in history, belief in a circular earth was dismissed by "experts" as fantasy and even heresy, even though reasonable scientific evidence supported it. In my opinion one of the greatest impediments to advancement of the human condition is the opinion of "experts."

These early childhood experiences changed me. I became acutely more sensitive to the feelings of others. Throughout my youth I would often feel the pain and emotions of my friends, neighbors, and even complete strangers. This may have been the reason I never craved the company of others and preferred being alone or in nature. I thought this was something everyone experienced as my mother and father both had similar "gifts". I suspect that my brother (now deceased) and sister are also sensitive but, strangely enough, that topic has never been broached. It was not until I was in high school that I came to the realization that most people do not have these experiences. When I was fifteen my father died as the end result of several heart attacks and strokes. I was close to my father and emotionally shut down for about fifteen years. I did not want to feel anything ever again. For many years I was indifferent to both the existence of my own feelings as well as the feelings of others. It wasn't until I began medical school that I became reacquainted with the sensitivity to others that I experienced in my youth.

I was traditionally trained in the scientific method: a master's degree in microbiology from Roosevelt University (Chicago) under the tutelage of Laura Bradford PhD; a PhD in immunology from Northwestern University (Chicago) under the guidance of a tremendous mentor, Byung Kim PhD. My medical training at Rush University Medical School in Chicago was instrumental to my learning how pathological processes occur, resulting in chronic illness. Early in my medical career I recognized most of the common medical systems, traditional and nontraditional, by themselves were incomplete. It was as if thousands of years ago a complete medical/healing system was taken apart and strewn to the four corners of the world. Over the centuries, different peoples have discovered some the pieces of this complete healing system and assumed that each piece by itself was the answer to illness and disease.

Little of what I learned in medical school and residency addressed the role the mind and spirit play in illness and healing. Indeed, the importance of the mind was dismissed or at best attributed to the great "black box" of the placebo effect. The role of the spirit was NEVER discussed in my medical training. It was something best left for the clergy and was not to be pursued by "serious" physicians and scientists. I began to realize that chronic illness is the result of the interplay between the body, mind, and spirit (add karma if you believe in karma, which I do). Karma is believed to be a spiritual principle of cause and effect. The actions of an individual in one lifetime can influence the experiences, including health, of an individual in a future lifetime. Conversely, healing and true health can only be achieved by treating the body, mind, and spirit together, i.e., to see them as three interconnected parts of the whole. I wanted to understand how the body, mind, and spirit interacted, resulting in either illness or health. Having experienced part of the spiritual world as a child, I recognized that the mind and spirit play important roles in the chronic illness of the body. I needed many more tools than traditional medicine had to offer. Fortunately in 2000 Andrew Weil MD began his fellowship program in integrative medicine at the University of Arizona. A fellowship is an in-depth program of learning beyond medical school and residency. Fellowships take one or more years to complete. Integrative medicine is the combination of the best of traditional and nontraditional medicine. I graduated with the inaugural class in 2002.

Even after fellowship training in integrative medicine, I felt that I was still missing an important aspect of healing. I needed more understanding and training in psychic healing techniques, also known as bio-energy healing. The results of my early attempts with energy-based healing were highly variable. Sometimes I would hit a home run and other times simply strike out. I could not find a reason for such variability. Like major league baseball players, my success average was about 280. I wanted to bat 1000. Psychic healing or bio-energy healing is not taught in medical schools so I had to seek out teachers who could enlighten me with a deeper understanding and more efficient healing techniques. That was surprisingly difficult. Although there are people in this world who are quite proficient at bio-energy healing, learning directly from them can be a hit-or-miss proposition since they have not created a specific school or curriculum. In order to be proficient as a bio-energy healer, an alchemic-like transformation of the practitioner must occur. A practitioner must become a good conduit for the flow of energy. This does not happen with a weekend seminar or multi-day certification course. It takes time, dedication, and curiosity. In ancient times, these spiritual teachings would be taught at specific locations such as the temple at Delphi in Greece, the Shaolin temple in China, and the numerous mystery schools of ancient Egypt. After much searching and trials, I discovered a school where this is taught in a structured program with care and wisdom. After several years of study I earned my doctorate in metaphysical studies at Delphi University in the tiny town of McCaysville in northern Georgia. So this is where I am today, a traditionally trained scientist and medical physician integrating many nontraditional therapies and approaches including energy-based healing into a more complete medical approach for treating chronic illness and promoting a state of health.

Let me emphasize that EVERYONE has the ability to heal themselves and participate in the healing of others. It is not just limited to a select few miracle workers like in ancient times. Everyone can perform miracles. It is part of our heritage as human beings and it is our strongest connection to all of our brothers and sisters. That means today there are seven billion potential healers on the earth-you, me, and everyone else. Sir Isaac Newton once said, *"If I have seen further than others, it is by standing upon the shoulders of giants."* The statement holds true for me, and for all of us. If you have read this book, I congratulate you because this means that you are already waking up to your own unrestricted potential, and that my sisters and brothers is, without any doubt, the greatest miracle of all.

BIBLIOGRAPHY

1. http://www.cdc.gov/chronicdisease/overview/
2. Ward BW, Schiller JS, Goodman RA. Multiple chronic conditions among U.S. adults: a 2012 update. *Prev Chronic Dis.* 2014;11:130389.
3. www.milkininstitute.com
4. Humphreys, Blodgett, Wagner (2014). "Estimating the efficacy of Alcoholics Anonymous without self-selection bias: an instrumental variables re-analysis of randomized clinical trials." *Alcoholism: Clinical and Experimental Research* 38 (11): 2688–94.
5. Marc Galanter, Zoran Josipovic, Helen Dermatis, Jochen Weber, and Mary Alice Millard (2016). "An initial fMRI study on neural correlates of prayer in members of Alcoholics Anonymous." *The American Journal of Drug and Alcohol Abuse.* doi: http://www.tandfonline.com/doi/full/10.3109/00952990.2016.1141912#abstract
6. http://www.ars.usda.gov/is/timeline/nutrition.htm
7. http://www.whale.to/a/light.html
8. Park YM, Steck SE, Fung TT, Zhang J, Hazlett LJ, Han K, Merchant AT. Mediterranean diet and mortality risk in metabolically healthy obese and metabolically unhealthy obese phenotypes. *Int J Obes (Lond).* 2016 Jun 24. [Epub ahead of print].
9. Alcubierre N, Martinez-Alonso M, Valls J, Rubinat E, Traveset A, Hernández M, Martínez-González MD, Granado-Casas M, Jurjo C, Vioque J, Navarrete-Muñoz EM, Mauricio D. Relationship of the adherence to the Mediterranean diet with health-related quality of life and treatment satisfaction in patients with type 2 diabetes mellitus: a post-hoc analysis of a cross-sectional study. Health Qual Life Outcomes. 2016 May 4;14(1):69.
10. Hardy Jr GE. The Burden of Chronic Disease: The Future is Prevention: Introduction to Dr. James Marks' presentation. Prev Chronic Dis. 2004 Apr; 1(2): A04.
11. https://www.nobelprize.org/nobel_prizes/medicine/laureates/1962/

12. *More than a chicken, fewer than a grape. Exact tally of human genes remains elusive.* Tina Hessman Saey. News Genes & Cells, Body & Brain. Vol. 178 #10, November 6, 2010, p. 5.

13. https://www.genome.gov/10001772/all-about-the--human-genome-project-hgp/

14. http://www.nhlbi.nih.gov/health/health-topics/topics/sca

15. http://www.nhlbi.nih.gov/health/health-topics/topics/cf

16. https://www.genome.gov/10001220/learning-about-taysachs-disease/

17. https://en.wikipedia.org/wiki/Epigenomics

18. William Shakespeare, *The Merchant of Venice.* Act III, Scene V.

19. Dusek JA, Otu HH, Wohlhueter AL, Bhasin M, Zerbini LF, Joseph MG, Benson H, Libermann TA Genomic counter-stress changes induced by the relaxation response. PLoS One. 2008 Jul 2;3(7):e2576.

20. Saatcioglu F. Regulation of gene expression by yoga, meditation and related practices: a review of recent studies. Asian J Psychiatr. 2013 Feb;6(1):74-7.

21. Bower JE, Irwin MR. Mind-body therapies and control of inflammatory biology: A descriptive review. Brain Behav Immun. 2015 Jun 23.

22. Piatigorsky J, O'Brien WE, Norman BL, Kalumuck K, Wistow GJ, Borras T, Nickerson JM, Wawrousek EF. "Gene sharing by delta-crystallin and argininosuccinate lyase." Proc Nat Acad Sci USA. 1988. May; 85 (10): 3479–83.

23. Conklin Q, King B, Zanesco A, Pokorny J, Hamidi A, Lin J, Epel E, Blackburn E, Saron C. Telomere lengthening after three weeks of an intensive insight meditation retreat. Psychoneuroendocrinology. 2015 Nov;61:26-7.

24. Schutte NS, Malouff JM. A meta-analytic review of the effects of mindfulness meditation on telomerase activity. Psychoneuroendocrinology. 2014 Apr;42:45-8.

25. Schrauf, R. W., & Sanchez, J. (2011). The shifting structure of emotion semantics across immigrant generations: Effects of the second culture on the first. In M. Schmid & W. Lowie (Eds.) *Modeling bilingualism: From*

structure to chaos (pp. 177-198). Amsterdam, Philadelphia: John Benjamins.

26. National Association for Sport and Physical Education. *The Fitness Equation: Physical Activity + Balanced Diet = Fit Kids.* Reston, VA: National Association for Sport and Physical Education, 1999.

27. U.S. Department of Health and Human Services. *Healthy People 2010.* Less than half the older adult population is physically active (Centers for Disease Control and Prevention. *CDC Behavioral Risk Factor Surveillance Survey.* http://www.cdc.gov/brfss/)

28. U.S. Department of Health and Human Services. *Healthy People 2020.*